Clinics in Human Lactation

Achieving Exclusive Breastfeeding: Translating Research into Action

Miriam Labbok, MD, MPH, IBCLC

Emily Taylor, MPH, CD (DONA)

Kathy Parry, MPH, IBCLC

Exclusive Breastfeeding is Achievable: Translating Research into Action Planning

Miriam Labbok, MD, MPH, IBCLC

Emily Taylor, MPH, CD (DONA)

Kathy Parry, MPH, IBCLC

Praeclarus Press, LLC

2504 Sweetgum Lane

Amarillo, Texas 79124 USA

806-367-9950

www.PraeclarusPress.com

DISCLAIMER

The information contained in this publication is advisory only and is not intended to replace sound clinical judgment or individualized patient care. The author disclaims all warranties, whether expressed or implied, including any warranty as the quality, accuracy, safety, or suitability of this information for any particular purpose.

ISBN: 978-1-939807-83-0

Foreword

"Achieving Exclusive Breastfeeding in the United States: Findings and Recommendations" was prepared for the United States Breastfeeding Committee (USBC) in 2007/8 and published in 2009. While the USBC was the sponsoring organization, the funding was provided by the United States Department of Health and Human Services. It was written by Miriam Labbok, MD, MPH, Professor of Maternal and Child Health and Director, the Carolina Global Breastfeeding Institute (CGBI) and Emily Taylor, MPH, then a graduate student at the University of North Carolina (UNC) School of Public Health, and now Senior Projects Director at the Institute. This update and revision builds on that paper and previous and subsequent work by the authors, and includes additional resources, attention to subsequent breastfeeding research and advocacy, and consideration of program activity that has occurred in subsequent years. Permission to update this paper was obtained from the USBC Leadership Team.

The increase in published research on exclusive breastfeeding issues encouraged this revision, update, and expansion, and permission was obtained from the USBC Leadership Team to proceed, based on the original constructs. New elements were designed by Emily Taylor, and the update in the annotated bibliography and related text was facilitated by Kathy Parry, a new member of the CGBI team. In addition to presenting the updated research annotations, this revision highlights promising activities and programs in the United States that are helping eliminate identified barriers to achieving exclusive breastfeeding.

The cover of this book does not show the face of the woman who is breastfeeding, and too often lactation experts become so involved with the baby, that we forget that it is the mother who primarily needs our support to obtain unbiased information and to succeed in her breastfeeding decisions. We dedicate this book to all the women whose faces we do not know, but who will hopefully benefit from the actions that you – the readers – will take, based on the information herein.

We welcome comment, discussion, and most of all, *action* towards the achievement of exclusive breastfeeding in the U.S., Europe, and beyond.

Table of Contents

Chapter 1. Introduction

The Need to Advance Exclusive Breastfeeding: The Changing Environment of Support for Exclusive Breastfeeding

Breastfeeding is the only infant and young child feeding approach, and human milk is the only food fully adapted to the physiology of human infants (Jones, Steketee, Black, Bhutta, & Morris, 2003; World Health Organization/UNICEF, 2003). Optimal breastfeeding is defined as initiation of breastfeeding immediately after birth (WHO/UNICEF, 1989), exclusively breastfeeding until six months of infant age, and continuation of breastfeeding with age-appropriate complementary foods and feeding up to two years of age or longer (World Health Organization/UNICEF, 2003). The World Health Organization and UNICEF support this pattern of infant and young child feeding because there is evidence that this pattern is associated with optimal maternal and child health outcomes.

What is Exclusive Breastfeeding?

The World Health Organization defines exclusive breastfeeding (EBF) as providing infants with only "breast milk from the mother or a wet nurse, or expressed breast milk, and no other liquids or solids, with the exception of drops or syrups consisting of vitamins, mineral supplements, or medicines" (World Health Organization, 1991). Exclusive breastfeeding differs from predominant breastfeeding (PBF), wherein human milk constitutes infants' primary nutritional source, but infants are also given other liquids, such as water, tea, juices, oral rehydration salt solutions, or ritual fluids. Other definitions in the literature and in use by some researchers also differentiate between exclusive breastfeeding and exclusive human milk feeding. This is especially important for the study of anatomy, physiology, and health responses, since the impact on both mother and child differ with milk expression and storage, and feeding of expressed milk by bottle and cup when compared to the anatomy, physiology, and health responses to direct breastfeeding (Labbok & Krasovec, 1990).

Why is it Important to Support Exclusive Breastfeeding?

Exclusive breastfeeding is the most effective global public health intervention for child survival (Darmstadt et al., 2005; Jones et al., 2003; World Health Organization/UNICEF, 2003). Therefore, while any breastfeeding is physiologically normal for optimal health outcomes (Ip et al., 2007), early initiation and exclusive breastfeeding for the first six months are optimal because of the resultant infant and child survival, growth, and development and improved maternal health (Edmond et al., 2006; Raisler, Alexander, & O'Campo, 1999). Human milk provides all of the nutrient requirements for infants less than six months of age, about half of their energy requirement from six to 12 months, and approximately one third their energy requirement throughout the child's second year of life (World Health Organization, 2000-2004). Human milk also includes all of the water, vitamins, minerals, carbohydrates, fats, proteins, digestive enzymes, and hormones that a developing child needs (Emmett & Rogers, 1997). The specific composition of human milk varies during each feed, throughout each day, and as the child ages, accommodating changing needs and providing the specific nutrients needed from the mothers' intake and stores. Human milk also provides immuno-protective factors for infants, selectively recruiting valuable antibodies and other factors from the mother.

Commercial infant formula manufacturers may attempt to replicate the nutritional components of human milk; however, there are literally hundreds of factors in human milk that cannot be reproduced, and others that cannot be successfully incorporated into a commercially viable human milk substitute (Labbok, Clark, & Goldman, 2004). Breastfeeding provides both a food and a physiologically based interaction between two individuals whereby both achieve a healthy, normal hormonal and biological milieu. This normalization of maternal postpartum physiology may be the underlying reason why breastfeeding is associated with lowered maternal risk of breast and ovarian cancers (Ip et al., 2007). EBF also contributes to cost-effective birth spacing. Hence, the use of any commercial infant feeding substitutes increases the drain on family and population health and other resources. A few studies have attempted to assess the costs and savings associated with exclusive breastfeeding. It has been estimated that breastfeeding costs approximately $600 annually in additional foods for the mother, whereas the cost of commercial formula alone, without bottles and other related paraphernalia, is approximately $1500 annually (in 1997 dollars, or $2150 in 2013 dollars, as per U.S. Department of Labor CPI index conversion; Montgomery & Splett, 1997). On a population level, research demonstrates that commercial formula feeding increases healthcare spending by $331-$475 per never-breastfed infant in the first year of life (Ball & Bennett, 2001). Cost savings analyses suggest that $13 billion in healthcare costs could be saved if breastfeeding rates were to increase to the *Healthy People 2010* objectives (Bartick & Reinhold, 2010).

Finally, there are environmental costs with the use of human milk substitutes, often referred to as 'breastmilk substitutes' or BMS. In 1991, it was reported that 86,000 tons of tin and 1,230 tons of paper were consumed in the packaging of formula annually (Radford, 1992). The production of the formula itself causes unnecessary damage to and consumption of environmental resources (Labbok, 1994), such as dairy industry waste, deforestation, soil erosion, pesticide contamination, and water pollution. One recent analysis concluded that the contribution to the carbon footprint of formula use in the United States is comparable to running 50,000 cars for a year (Tinling, 2011).

Which Organizations and Policies Support Exclusive Breastfeeding?

There is worldwide consensus that optimal infant feeding includes exclusive breastfeeding for the first six months of life. This is supported by expert opinions, such as those expressed by the World Health Organization (World Health Organization/UNICEF, 2003), UNICEF (2012), United States Department of Health and Human Services (2000), United States Agency for International Development (2012), American Academy of Pediatrics (Eidelman et al., 2012), American Academy of Family Physicians (2008), Academy of Breastfeeding Medicine (Liebert, 2008), American Dietetic Association (James & Lessen, 2009), American College of Obstetricians and Gynecologists (2007), American College of Preventive Medicine (2012), National Association of Pediatric Nurse Practitioners (2001), and others.

In addition to widespread support among national and international health organizations, national governments, including the U.S., reinforce the importance of supporting optimal breastfeeding by developing encouraging policies and objectives. While countries that offer national healthcare generally include breastfeeding support within the extant services, in countries like the United States, where there is no national system of healthcare provision, it remains the option of the individual and/ or insurance companies to seek coverage for breastfeeding support. The 2010 Affordable Care Act (ACA) for the first time legislates that employers provide workplace accommodations that allow women to express their milk in a location, other than a restroom, that is private and clean (U.S. Department of Labor, 2010). However, this is restricted to hourly wage earners in companies that have at least 50 employees, eliminating this protection for a large proportion of workers.

U.S. Surgeon General Regina Benjamin released an unprecedented document from the nation's highest medical office in January 2011. The *Surgeon General's Call to Action to Support Breastfeeding* urges the nation's healthcare providers, employers, insurers, policymakers, researchers, and community at large to work toward removing the barriers to breastfeeding (U.S. Department of Health and Human Services, 2011). The Health Goals for the United States are outlined in *Healthy People 2020*. In support of *Healthy People 2020* goals, the U.S. Surgeon General's Office aims to increase current rates of exclusive breastfeeding from 35% to 46.2% at three months, and from 14.8% to 25.5% at six months by 2020 (U.S. Department of Health and Human Services, 2010).

The Innocenti Declaration on the Protection, Promotion and Support of Breastfeeding was produced and adopted at the WHO/UNICEF policymakers' meeting, "Breastfeeding in the 1990s: A Global Initiative" (1990) and signed by Dr. Audrey Nora, formerly Chief of the MCHB/ HRSA/DHHS. It envisions "an environment that enables mothers, families, and other caregivers to make informed decisions about optimal feeding and provides the skilled support needed to achieve the highest attainable standard of health and development for infants and young children" (UNICEF, 2005). The declaration called for the creation or reinforcement of a "breastfeeding culture," which requires a strong rejection of "bottle-feeding culture." Those present at the meeting believed that this could occur through social mobilization led by societal leaders from multiple venues. Four operational targets were established for member nations (UNICEF/WHO, 1990):

- Appoint a national breastfeeding coordinator with appropriate authority, and establish a multi-sectoral national breastfeeding committee composed of representatives from relevant government departments, non-governmental organizations, and health professional associations.

- Ensure that every facility providing maternity services fully practices all the Ten Steps to Successful Breastfeeding set out in the WHO/UNICEF statement on breastfeeding and maternity services.

- Give effect to the principles and aim of the *International Code of Marketing of Breast-milk Substitutes* and subsequent relevant Health Assembly resolutions in their entirety.

- Enact imaginative legislation protecting the breastfeeding rights of working women.

These were expanded in the new millennium in the *Global Strategy for Infant and Young Child Feeding* to include five additional operational targets:

- Develop, implement, monitor, and evaluate a comprehensive policy on infant and young child feeding, in the context of national policies and programs for nutrition, child, and reproductive health, and poverty reduction.

- Ensure that the health and other relevant sectors protect, promote, and support exclusive breastfeeding for six months and continued breastfeeding up to two years of age or beyond, while providing women access to the support they require – in the family, community, and workplace – to achieve this goal.

- Promote timely, adequate, safe, and appropriate complementary feeding with continued breastfeeding.

- Provide guidance on feeding infants and young children in exceptionally difficult circumstances, and on the related support required by mothers, families, and other caregivers.

- Consider what new legislation or other suitable measures may be required, as part of a comprehensive policy on infant and young child feeding, to give effect to the principles and aim of the *International Code of Marketing of Breast-Milk Substitutes* and to subsequent relevant Health Assembly resolutions.

The 30 countries present at the Innocenti meeting pledged to achieve the four operational targets by 1995. Although few today have fully implemented these four operational targets, let alone the additional targets in the *Global Strategy*, several factor have emerged, not the least of which is steady attention to child survival, that continually bring the discussion back to breastfeeding.

Breastfeeding is Back!

The increased interest in breastfeeding as a vital health intervention has stimulated social and political response in many parts of the world. In the U.S., the Surgeon General's 2011 *Call to Action to Support Breastfeeding* (U.S. Department of Health and Human Services, 2011) builds on the support for exclusive breastfeeding expressed by virtually all health professional associations. In Europe, the 2004 *Blueprint for Action on Breastfeeding* (Cattaneo, 2004), the Baby-Friendly Initiative (BFI), and related activities in the UK (UNICEF UK, 2012) reflect this growing reality. These examples from industrialized country settings illustrate the recognition that the breastfeeding norm has been lost, and therefore it may be necessary to observe and seek ideas for solutions from settings that have retained a breastfeeding norm, such as selected developing country settings. It is often the industrialization, *per se*, that serves as a contextual barrier to breastfeeding; the dependence on attendance at a workplace in order to be a viable part of the economy can in and of itself create contextual and physical obstacles and constraints to breastfeeding.

Globally, breastfeeding has become more socially and politically acceptable today due to a continuum of global efforts, initially stimulated by attention to the marketing practices of infant formula manufacturers. Nearly 80 years ago, Dr. Cicely Williams' call for attention to bottle-baby deaths was marked by a presentation to the Singapore Rotary Club. Using the title *Milk and Murder,* she said, *"misguided propaganda on infant feeding should be punished as the most criminal form of sedition, and that those deaths should be regarded as murder."* Later, in 1968, Dr. Derrick Jelliffe coined the term *"commerciogenic malnutrition"* to describe the impact of industry marketing practices on infant health (Jelliffe 1972). The recognition that there are risks with formula use also heightened the need to revitalize support for the individual skills associated with successful breastfeeding.

This breadth of support is strengthened by the increase in published research showing that breastfeeding, especially exclusive breastfeeding (EBF) during the first six months of life, is strongly associated with optimal health outcomes for mother and child in both the short and long term. However, this practice remains a rarity, adopted by the minority of families worldwide. The result is that duration of breastfeeding, in general, and exclusive breastfeeding, in particular, continue to be well below the World Health Organization recommendations, and in the U.S., below the *Healthy People 2020* objectives.

What are the Trends in Exclusive Breastfeeding Rates Worldwide and in the U.S.?

Recent available exclusive breastfeeding data are presented in Table 1.1 below. Trend analysis from 1990 – 2004 indicate an annual average increase of one-half of one percentage points, while a similar analysis, with more countries, from 1995-2008 and to 2010, indicate an average annual increase only slightly less. Therefore, the rate of exclusive breastfeeding rate worldwide in the first six months of life may be rising at a minimally slower rate in the last few years (Labbok, 2012). However, given the differences in these analyses, it is very difficult to discern any changes in the rate of increase over shorter periods of time. The data in Table 1.1 illustrate these trend analyses in a single table, where the 1990/2004 data are based on a subset of 37 countries, covering 60% of the developing world's population (*Innocenti +15* publication using UNICEF 2005 data). The 1995/2010 data are based on a subset of 77 countries with trend data, covering 70% of births in the developing world. Latin America and the Caribbean were excluded due to insufficient data coverage. Regional trends indicate an increase from 30 to 46%, excluding Brazil and Mexico (http://www. childinfo.org/breastfeeding_progress.html; UNICEF global databases 2011, from Multiple Indicator Cluster Surveys (MICS), Demographic Health Surveys (DHS) and other national surveys). All of these estimates 1) are based on data gathered over a period of time greater than the single year indicated, 2) exclude China, and 3) are based on data sets that have insufficient data for countries in South and Central America. The latest figures indicate that the rate of EBF in the developing world is about 39% (UNICEF, 2012).

Table 1.1. Exclusive Breastfeeding Rates Among Infants in the First Six Months of Life, by Region and by Year.

Region	1990	1995*	2004	2008*	2010*
Central/Eastern Europe, Commonwealth of Independent States		9		29	30
East Asia Pacific	39	27	38	30	31
Eastern/Southern Africa	34	33	48	46	49
South Asia	43	41	47	45	45
Middle East/North Africa	30	35	38	32	34
Western/Central Africa	4	14	22	24	24
Overall for Developing Countries	34	32	41	39	39

Note: The 1990 and 2004 estimates are not directly comparable with the 1995 and 2008 data nor the 2010 data, as each published study (see sources in text) included different sub-sets of countries; however, they are presented with description for readers' consideration. **Sources:** (further described in the text) *Innocenti +15* publication; http://www.childinfo. org/breastfeeding_progress.html; and UNICEF, 2012.

This may be viewed as both positive and negative: every percentage point increase saves lives and reduces suffering. *The State of the World's Children* noted that exclusive breastfeeding rates increased by nearly 20% in the decade of the 1990s (UNICEF, 2002). Child Info reports a similar or greater increase in the last decade for 23 countries; however, trends for the decade overall are not presented (UNICEF). The progress may be directly attributable to the UNICEF/WHO leadership in 1990. They increased attention to the issue and defined the need for action in the *Innocenti Declaration* operational targets: National policy, authority, and commitment; implementation of the Ten Steps for Breastfeeding Support in maternity settings; legislation of the *International Code of Marketing of Breast-milk Substitutes* and subsequent World Health Assembly resolutions; and workplace accommodation, including paid maternity leave and paid breaks to allow breastfeeding during the workday for both formal and informal work situations (UNICEF/WHO, 1990).

U.S. data show that while about 75% of infants are initially breastfed in the U.S., exclusive breastfeeding is practiced at three months by 33.5% of mother/baby dyads, and at six months by 13.8%, while the 2020 objectives are 46.2% and 25.5%, respectively (DHHS Centers for Disease Control and Prevention, 2012). According to the CDC's *Breastfeeding Report Card*, California and Vermont are the only two states in the U.S. meeting the *Healthy People 2020* objectives for exclusive breastfeeding at six months (Centers for Disease Control and Prevention, 2011a). However, it is important to recognize that there is great variability in these rates among several socioeconomic and geographic groupings (see Table 1.2 and Figure 1.1).

Figure 1.1. Any and Exclusive Breastfeeding Rates in Percent by Age Among Children Born in 2007.

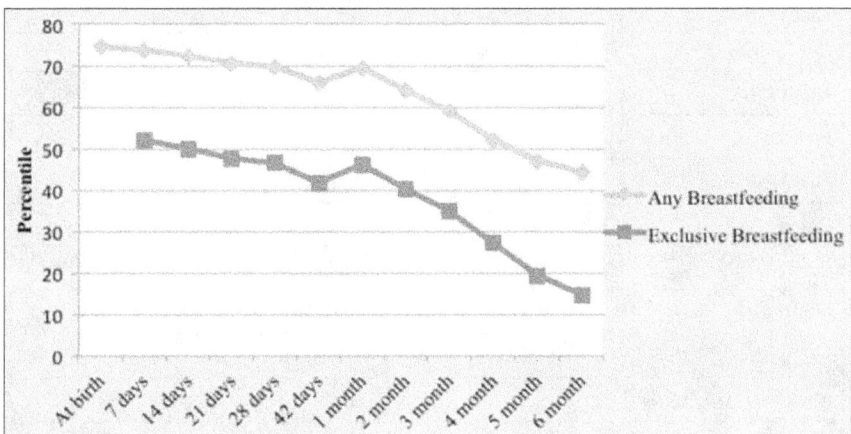

Source: National Immunization Survey, Centers for Disease Control and Prevention, Department of Health and Human Services, 2012.

Table 1.2. Breastfeeding Rates by Socio-Demographic Factors Among Children Born in 2007 (Percent +/- half 95% Confidence Interval).

Socio-demographic Factors	Ever	Exclusive Breast-feeding1	Exclusive Breast-feeding1
	Breastfeeding	Through 3 Months	Through 6 Months
2020 Goals	81.9	46.2	25.5
U.S. National	75.0±1.2	33.0±1.2	13.3±0.9
Sex			
Male	75.4±1.6	33.1±1.7	12.9±1.2
Female	74.6±1.7	32.9±1.8	13.7±1.3
Race/Ethnicity			
American Indian or Alaska Native	73.8±6.9	27.6±7.3	13.2±6.3
Asian or Pacific Islander	83.0±5.2	34.1±6.0	14.5±4.3
-Asian	86.4±5.7	34.5±6.6	16.8±5.2
-Native Hawaiian and other	72.4±11.1	31.0±11.8	6.5±3.9
Black or African American	59.7±2.9	22.7±2.4	8.2±1.5
White	77.7±1.2	35.3±1.4	14.4±1.0
Hispanic or Latino	80.6±2.4	33.4±3.0	13.4±2.2
Not Hispanic or Latino (NH)	72.8±1.3	32.9±1.3	13.2±0.9
-NH Black or African American	58.1±3.1	21.9±2.5	8.0±1.5
-NH White	76.2±1.4	35.8±1.5	14.8±1.0
Birth Order			
First Born	74.5±1.6	33.4±1.7	13.8±1.2
Not First Born	75.6±1.6	32.6±1.8	12.6±1.2
Receiving WIC2			
Yes	67.5±1.8	25.5±1.8	9.2±1.2
No, but eligible	77.5±4.7	39.9±5.6	19.2±4.8
Ineligible	84.6±1.4	41.9±1.8	17.7±1.3
Maternal Age, Years			
<20	59.7±7.9	18.1±6.4	7.9±4.7
20-29	69.7±2.1	28.8±2.1	10.2±1.3
>=30	79.3±1.4	36.6±1.6	15.5±1.2

Maternal Education			
Not a High School Graduate	67.0±3.4	23.7±3.3	9.2±2.3
High School Graduate	66.1±2.5	25.8±2.5	8.9±1.5
Some College	76.5±2.1	34.1±2.5	14.4±2.1
College Graduate	88.3±1.1	45.9±1.9	19.6±1.4
Maternal Marital Status			
Married	81.7±1.3	39.0±1.5	16.7±1.2
Unmarried[3]	61.3±2.4	20.9±2.2	6.4±1.2
Residence			
MSA[4], Central City	75.5±1.8	32.8±2.0	13.3±1.3
MSA, Non-Central City	77.9±1.7	34.9±2.0	13.9±1.5
Non-MSA	66.4±2.9	28.8±2.4	11.8±1.7
Poverty Income Ratio[5], %			
<100%	67.0±2.7	25.0±2.7	8.6±1.7
100%-184%	71.2±2.8	31.7±3.0	12.7±2.1
185%-349%	77.7±2.4	36.0±2.5	14.6±1.7
≥350%	84.4±1.7	41.1±2.1	17.6±1.6

[1]Exclusive breastfeeding is defined as ONLY human milk — No solids, no water, and no other liquids

[2]WIC = Special Supplemental Nutrition Program for Women, Infants, and Children.

[3]Unmarried includes never married, widowed, separated, divorced.

[4]MSA = Metropolitan Statistical Area defined by the Census Bureau.

[5]Poverty Income Ratio = Ratio of self-reported family income to the federal poverty threshold value depending on the number of people in the household.

Source: National Immunization Survey, Centers for Disease Control and Prevention, Department of Health and Human Services, 2012.

Married women are exclusively breastfeeding at six months nearly three times as often as unmarried women (16.7% vs. 6.4%). Rates of exclusive breastfeeding at six months increase as maternal age increases: from about 8% of mothers under 20 years of age, to 15.5% among mothers older than 30. Socioeconomic status, nationality, race/ethnicity, and maternal educational attainment are also strongly associated with initiation and duration of exclusive breastfeeding (Kurinij & Shiono, 1991; Ludvigsson & Ludvigsson, 2005). Exclusive breastfeeding rates at six months for Whites, Asian or Pacific Islanders, American Indian, and Hispanic/Latinos are about 13-14%. However, the rate found for African-American women is notably lower, at 8.2%. African-Americans also have far lower initiation rates than any other racial/ethnic groupings, at 59.7%. Rates also vary by location, suggesting that there are additional local social influences on exclusive breastfeeding practices. The Southeastern region of the country generally has the lowest rate, while the Northwest has the highest.

It is possible that governmental programs also impact exclusive breastfeeding. For example, mothers who are not enrolled in WIC, whether they are eligible or not, are nearly two times as likely to exclusively breastfeed to six months as WIC-enrolled mothers (9.2% vs. 17.7-19.2%). Family and maternal income are correlated with EBF, with families with higher incomes demonstrating higher rates of EBF initiation and duration (Li, Fridinger, & Grummer-Strawn, 2002). However, the association of WIC and lower rates of exclusive breastfeeding is not attributable to income alone; women eligible for, but not enrolled in WIC demonstrate rates of breastfeeding similar to women of higher income brackets. The rate of exclusive breastfeeding drops off more rapidly than the rate of any breastfeeding, especially during the period of four to six months of age (Figure 1.1).

EBF rates are lower among several sub-populations of U.S. women: non-Hispanic Black mothers, those living in the South, those enrolled in WIC, those who are unmarried, younger age, low wealth, rurality, lower educational attainment, indicating multiple, perhaps interactive, mediating factors. However, as we will discuss, this does not mean that any one individual who falls within any one of these groupings necessarily breastfeeds accordingly. Rather, the take-home message is that on average there may be differences that merit consideration, and that efforts to decrease inequity and reduce disparities should consider the population that is being served by the intervention, but also should consider that the final breastfeeding decision and action is taken by the individual. Therefore, any exploration, translation, innovative intervention, or replication/scale-up must constantly consider what is known about the groupings, but also must consider each individual.

Planning for Action: Influence and Timing, and the 'E-TIERS' Approach

This book uses an innovation approach to address the primary issue of increasing exclusive breastfeeding, starting with the issue – exclusive breastfeeding (EBF). We then fully explore and translate findings using two constructs. The first includes major areas, or disciplines, where intervention might most closely impact the environments in which women and families are making and implementing their infant feeding decisions: Healthcare; Social, Workplace, and Political/Policy; and Media and Marketing. The second construct is that of the Lifecycle and Timing – there are different interventions that may be most important at different times.

The third construct is the underlying approach used in this book to address the issue of exclusive breastfeeding and its support. This is a relatively new construct designed to utilize a transdisciplinary approach that continually forces consideration of multiple components of the issue in question: the **E-TIERS** approach. First, we EXPLORE what is known both by reviewing the literature and by going beyond this, exploring ongoing programs and initiatives. In our exploration we followed a previously established construct for identifying issues by both identified time periods and by area that most impact a mother's environment: healthcare; social, workplace and political; and media and marketing. We then TRANSLATE these findings into recommendations for INNOVATIVE IMPLEMENTATION of an intervention, dissemination, or social change with ongoing monitoring of both processes and outcomes. We propose that any implementation be coupled with a plan to EVALUATE. The outcomes of evaluation must be used to adapt, modify, and improve in order to REPLICATE, reassess, adapt, then SUSTAINABLE SCALE-UP what works, so that more and more mothers are aware of the importance of their feeding behavior and experience in an environment that supports healthful behaviors.

These three constructs enabled us to go deeper into the socio-ecological framework, adding the dimensions of the timing of proposed innovative intervention in the lifecycle, as well as the type of intervention required. The findings and recommendations are discussed and presented in relation to the *Surgeon General's Call to Action to Support Breastfeeding*, which includes 20 action areas based on exploration of a socio-ecological framework, the European Blueprint, and the World Health Organization/UNICEF *Global Strategy for Infant and Young Child Feeding* (U.S. Department of Health and Human Services, 2011).

Chapter 2. Exploring the Areas of Influence

Obstacles and Opportunities for Exclusive Breastfeeding During Specific Time Periods in the Reproductive Health Continuum

Definitions: Influences and When They Might Have an Impact

Three primary areas of influence are often identified as providing obstacles to successful exclusive breastfeeding, but they may also offer opportunities. These include:

1. Healthcare systems and providers

2. Socioeconomic and sociopolitical factors

3. Media and marketing

The published literature addressing each of these areas is examined both to assess the impact they may have on achievement of exclusive breastfeeding, and how that impact might vary at different points in time during the continuum associated with exclusive breastfeeding decision-making and behaviors.

Eight potentially critical time periods were originally outlined by a USDHHS expert committee to assess influences on breastfeeding in general (Simopoulos & Grave, 1984). Table 2.1 identifies the time periods and explains what is happening during each period that might impact the mother's decision to exclusively breastfeed.

Table 2.1. Critical Times to Influence Mothers and the Mother-Child Dyad.

Time Period	Criticality: Rationale for Identification as a Critical Period for Exclusive Breast-feeding
Preconception / Inter-Conception	Knowledge development and planning by mother/family
Prenatal	Prospective counseling during period of high interest
Perinatal	Aspects of the birthing process influence breastfeeding initiation, continuation, and exclusivity

Immediate Postpartum Period	Establishment of the dyad; breastfeeding initiated
Days 3 – 12	Milk "comes in," adaptation following maternity discharge
Day 12 – Week 6	Establishment of mother/baby interaction and sufficiency of milk production
Weeks 6 – 12	Maintenance of sufficient milk production; period of maternal and infant physiological adaptations
Months 3 – 6	Drop-off in rates of EBF; adaptation to social influences and health worker inputs

Source: Simopoulos & Grave, 1984. Used with permission.

Figure 2.1. Contextual Framework illustrating the three primary sources of information and support for breastfeeding success. These, then, are the areas of influence where interventions may be most effective. Heavier lines in the schema indicate the possibility that greater influence may be associated with successful interventions at the specified time period during the reproductive cycle.

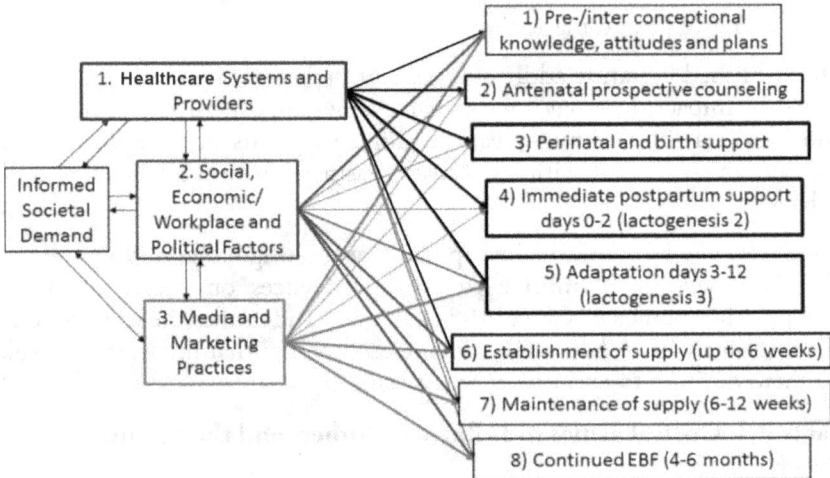

Source: USBC, 2008. Used with permission.

These primary sources of information are available to the mother and family at different periods of time throughout the reproductive life cycle. Each may have a greater or lesser impact, and be mediated by different pressures and concerns as is illustrated in Figure 2.2 below. Figure 2.2 offers an illustration of how the importance, or criticality, of each issue and the source of information might change with the differing time period under consideration. To better understand what is happening and where we should recommend intervention, it is important to consider the three dimensions of 1) Time, 2) Source, and 3) Criticality.

Figure 2.2. Potential Obstacles or Supports for Exclusive Breastfeeding by Eight Times in the Reproductive Continuum. The interventions and messages needed, as well as the target group for change, will vary across the continuum.

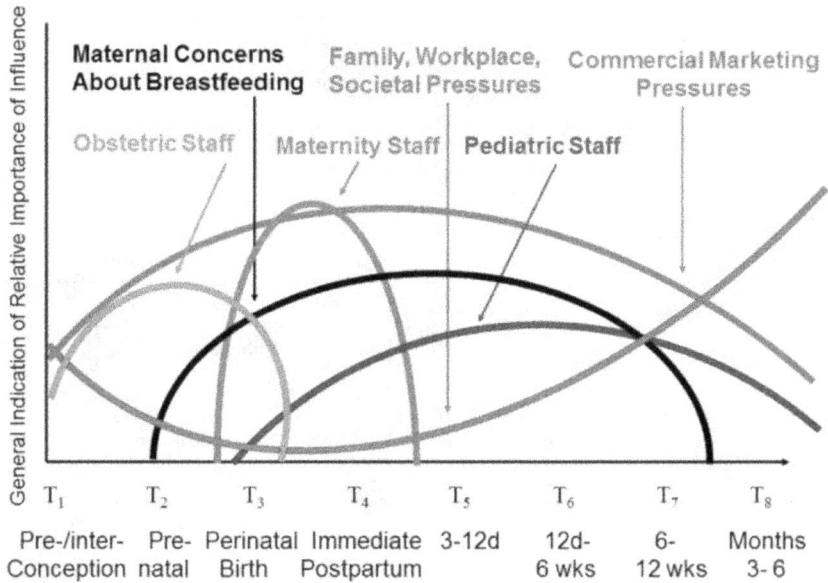

Source: Modified from USBC Publication, 2008. Used with permission.

Methods: Identification and Selection of Materials for Inclusion

The literature review included five components:

1) Searching the published literature for EBF-specific publications

2) Assessing the applicability of the evidence to this model and for the U.S.

3) Organizing evidence into the above-noted conceptual model and by timing of the potential intervention

4) Extrapolating themes and possible recommendations

5) Seeking review by those with experiential inputs

PUBMED and ASSIA search engines were employed, using broad-based search terms to maximize results. In addition, targeted searches using Google Scholar were used for more recent literature (see Table 2.2). The vast majority of studies identified and included in this review are studies from the United States and other industrialized countries. The few exceptions were included due to consistency of findings with those from industrialized settings.

Table 2.2. Search Terms

Exclusive breastfeeding OR Full Breastfeeding	
	+ Sociology
	+ Psychology
	+ Socioeconomic Status
	+ Maternal Factors
	+ Maternity Care
	+ Advertising
	+ Marketing Breastmilk Substitutes
	+ Time
	+ Healthcare Systems
	+ Hospital
	+ Birth
	+ Postpartum Support
	+ Lactation Consultants
	+ Nurse
	+ Midwife
	+ Obstetrician
	+ Pediatrician
	+ Policies
	+ Media
	+ Income
	+ Educational Attainment
	+ Demographics
	+ Analgesia
	+ Age
	+ Cesarean
	+ Epidural
	+ Pregnancy
	+ Preconception

	+ Bedsharing/cosleeping
	+ Employment
	+ Workplace
Additionally Targeted:	
	+ Antenatal Care
	+ BFHI/Baby Friendly
	+ Formula Advertising
	+ Lactation Support in Pediatric Offices
	+ Paid Maternity Leave
	+ Pediatrician Breastfeeding Education
	+ Peer Support
	+ NICU

Chapter 3. Findings

Obstacles, Opportunities, Current Interventions, and Gaps during Eight Time Periods in the Reproductive Health Cycle

Exploration that includes literature review, contacting experts, reading the grey literature, and keeping one's eyes open reveals that there have been many studies and programs designed to increase breastfeeding in general; many of these findings and approaches may impact the initiation and duration of *exclusive* breastfeeding. Therefore, an effort has been made to identify and summarize those studies and activities that are most likely to influence exclusivity. The findings on EBF are presented by time period in the reproductive life cycle, and include the three sets of factors explored: Health Services and Provider-Related Influences; Socioeconomic and Sociopolitical Influences; and Media and Marketing.

This presentation of findings includes the highlights gleaned from a review of the last 15-20 years of published literature and highlights recent findings that may be translated into intervention. Therefore, the demographic factors presented in the introduction are not highlighted, as they are not amenable to change. However, recognizing the demographic differences allows for targeting those populations who may be most in need of support with the interventions that emerge from this analysis.

We also include examples of extant interventions that impact breastfeeding decisions and practices, and that we believe may have a measurable impact on exclusive breastfeeding. These examples are presented throughout the findings as illustrations to reinforce research findings and to contribute to the full exploration needed to translate current knowledge into innovative implementable interventions.

Pre-/Inter-Conception

Women and their families may be very open to intervention during pre- and inter-conceptional times, especially those that target biomedical, behavioral, and social factors influencing health and pregnancy outcomes (Johnson et al., 2006). This is commonly a time when women and their immediate social networks are developing and planning parenting strategies, including plans to exclusively breastfeed (Lu et al., 2006; Moos, 2004).

Health Services and Provider-Related Influences on Exclusive Breastfeeding Pre- and Inter-Conception

Well-woman care during the pre- and inter-conceptional stages of women's lives typically occurs on an annual basis or less often. However, during pregnancy, the average middle-income woman sees her provider 13 times over 40 weeks (Binstock & Wolde-Tsadik, 1995). After birth, most healthcare interactions focus on well-child care (Moos, 2006). Since research suggests that women are highly receptive to health information as they plan their pregnancies, providers may be missing a valuable opportunity to educate women about the risks and benefits of infant feeding decisions (Scott, Landers, Hughes, & Binns, 2001). This is especially important, as women's preconceptional or inter-conceptional commitment to breastfeeding is positively associated with increased rates of EBF initiation and duration.

Socioeconomic and Sociopolitical Influences on Exclusive Breastfeeding Pre- and Inter-Conception

Studies have not focused on pre- or inter-conceptional exposure to social and political factors that may influence later exclusive breastfeeding. However, there is literature relevant to exclusive and continued breastfeeding that involves studying whether the pregnancy is intended, demographic factors, socioeconomic status, health beliefs and behaviors, and subsequent breastfeeding success.

Health education and beliefs have a demonstrated effect on rates of exclusive breastfeeding. First, maternal doubts about the benefits, feasibility, and adequacy of breastfeeding significantly affect EBF choices (Li, Darling, Maurice, Barker, & Grummer-Strawn, 2005; Li, Rock, & Grummer-Strawn, 2007); the more women know about exclusive breastfeeding before pregnancy, the more likely they are to practice it (Pechlivani et al., 2005). In addition, the source of the EBF information is important (Kronborg & Væth, 2004). Maternal, paternal, and maternal grandmother's attitudes regarding breastfeeding is positively associated with EBF (Li et al., 2005), and maternal empowerment and confidence predicts higher rates of EBF (Brown & Lee, 2011; Kronborg & Væth, 2004). Health behaviors such as smoking and over-nutrition are associated with later choice not to practice EBF (Hilson, Rasmussen, & Kjolhede, 2006; Li et al., 2005).

Media and Marketing Influences on Exclusive Breastfeeding Pre- and Inter-Conception

Studies on the impact of marketing of human milk substitutes during this period on later EBF have not been identified. However, we know women are increasingly exposed to advertisements; formula marketing data trends show that annual expenditures on advertisements grew from $29 million to over $46 million in the U.S. between 1999 and 2004 (U.S. Government

Accountability Office, 2006). The vast majority of advertisements in a recent study were found to violate the *International Code of Marketing of Breast-Milk Substitutes* (Alikaşşifoğglu et al., 2001). Breastfeeding promotion and education efforts cannot counteract this proliferation, as they are not supported by multi-million dollar advertising budgets. This greatly imbalanced presentation of information about infant feeding affects women's knowledge and attitudes about infant feeding, which arguably has measurable impact on later behaviors (Li et al., 2007). This is further supported by the documented influence of BF counseling in this period on subsequent rates of EBF (Anderson, Damio, Young, Chapman, & Perez-Escamilla, 2005; Chapman, Damio, Young, & Perez-Escamilla, 2004; Merten, Dratva, & Ackermann-Liebrich, 2005; Morrow et al., 1999). We know that the messages contained in formula advertisements are misleading to many women and undermine recommendations for exclusive breastfeeding (Parry, Taylor, Hall-Dardess, Walker, & Labbok, 2013). It is therefore important to ensure women have strong education in the benefits of breastfeeding and human milk and the risks of formula during the pre- and inter-conception time period, before women begin making infant feeding decisions.

Prenatal Period

Health System and Provider Influences on Exclusive Breastfeeding in the Prenatal Period

Women experience vastly increased frequency of exposure to healthcare providers, preventive health measures, and other forms of health education during the prenatal period and are likely to make positive health decisions and/or modify adverse health behaviors during this time (Institute for Clinical Systems Improvement, 2012; Verma, Chhatwal, & Varughese, 1995). The reported rate of women accessing prenatal care in the first trimester has steadily increased since 1990; however, comparisons over the last decade are impossible due to the 2003 change in the standard birth certificate that is gradually being adopted by U.S. states. Generally speaking, the vast majority of women in industrialized settings utilize prenatal care during their first trimester, with less than 10% waiting until the third trimester or not receiving any care at all (Martin et al., 2010; Martin et al., 2006). The majority of women experience 11 – 14 visits per pregnancy (DHHS *Healthy People 2010*, 2000). Prenatal care visits include multiple surveillance techniques designed for early identification of adverse pregnancy and birth outcomes, including sexually transmitted infection screening, testing fetuses for birth defects and proper growth and development, etc. Therefore, this is an important and appropriate time to maximize attention to the support of the development of the breastfeeding commitment. Evidence shows that attendance in a prenatal breastfeeding class is associated with higher EBF among women (Mistry, Freedman, Sweeney, & Hollenbeck, 2008; Semenic, Loiselle, & Gottlieb, 2008; Su et al., 2007; Tender et al., 2009; Whalen & Cramton, 2010).

Given the evidence that prenatal care can positively influence breastfeeding rates, health inequities in access to and use of prenatal care are arguably related to the disparities in breastfeeding rates (Yarmo & Malin, 2005). Figure 3.1 shows the differences by race in women receiving any care in the first trimester.

Figure 3.1. Women Receiving Any Care in the First Trimester, 2008.

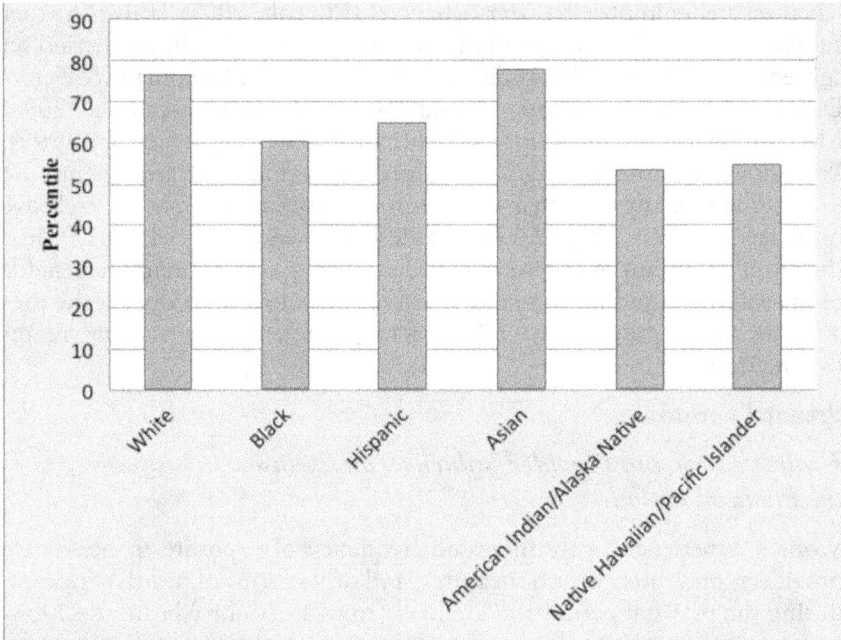

Source: Centers for Disease Control and Prevention. National Center for Health Statistics, National Vital Statistics System. Unpublished data. Analyzed by Maternal and Child Health Bureau and National Center for Health Statistics.

Figure 3.2 shows breastfeeding initiation and duration by race, with Hispanics having the highest rates and Blacks having the lowest.

Figure 3.2. Breastfeeding Initiation and Duration by Race.

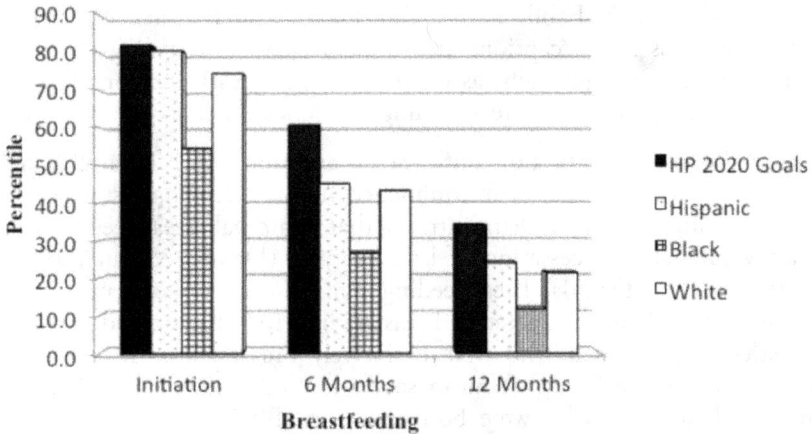

Source: Adapted from Centers for Disease Control and Prevention National Immunization Survey, Data from 2004-2008. (Centers for Disease Control, 2010).

Studies show that counseling pregnant women on the benefits and techniques of breastfeeding during prenatal visits is highly correlated with rates of EBF (Chapman et al., 2004; Verma et al., 1995). Additional opportunities for providers to positively impact EBF include counseling pregnant women on quitting smoking and attending a breastfeeding class (Whalen & Cramton, 2010). However, as surveillance practices increase, time spent on counseling is reportedly waning (Scott et al., 2001). Further, obstetricians, who attend the vast majority of births in the U.S., often fail to counsel their patients appropriately regarding EBF because they lack the necessary knowledge to do so (e.g., regarding milk production and BF techniques; Taveras et al., 2004). If the provider is able to provide culturally competent counseling, this has been associated with increased EBF (Yarmo & Malin, 2005). The United States Breastfeeding Committee has developed a list of evidence-based core competencies about breastfeeding that every healthcare provider should possess. This document is endorsed by 17 organizations, including the AAP (U.S. Breastfeeding Committee, 2010).

Social, Economic, and Political Influences on Exclusive Breastfeeding in the Prenatal Period

Many of the same social, economic, and political forces influencing EBF in the pre- and inter-conceptional periods continue to do so in the prenatal period, including knowledge and beliefs about the health rationale and ease-of-practice of EBF, career considerations, and health behaviors such as smoking and nutrition. This is a critical period for decision-making, so it is logical to hypothesize that perceived norms have significant impact on decision-making at this time. Evidence shows that intention to breastfeed is highly correlated with actual breastfeeding (Mistry et al., 2008), as well as exclusivity and duration (Bai, Middlestadt, Peng, & Fly, 2010; Dabritz, Hinton, & Babb, 2010). Additional research is needed on how best to address misperceptions and misconceptions regarding EBF and breastfeeding more generally, as these have been clearly demonstrated to have a negative impact on breastfeeding outcomes (Li et al., 2002).

Maternal empowerment and confidence is an important influence. Cindy Lee Dennis defines maternal confidence in breastfeeding using a self-efficacy framework and demonstrates that maternal breastfeeding self-efficacy predicts the cessation of breastfeeding (Dennis & Faux, 1999). Further use of Dennis' Breastfeeding Self-Efficacy Scale demonstrates an association between maternal breastfeeding self-efficacy and exclusive breastfeeding. Women who were exclusively breastfeeding in the study reported significantly higher mean scores for prenatal breastfeeding self-efficacy than those who were bottle feeding (Blyth et al., 2002). One study examining the relationship between breastfeeding outcomes and breastfeeding intentions, maternal self-efficacy, and maternal social support reveals that there is a strong and significant relationship between breastfeeding outcome and maternal self-efficacy that is mediated by a woman's intention to breastfeed. It also showed that the higher the degree of social support a woman receives, the higher the woman's self-efficacy, or breastfeeding confidence (Parkinson, Russell-Bennett, & Previte, 2010). Thus, social support can be seen as the ultimate driver of behavior:

Degree of Social Support > Maternal Self-Efficacy > Intention to Breastfeed > Breastfeeding Behavior

Media and Marketing Influences on Exclusive Breastfeeding in the Prenatal Period

Exposure to advertising for commercial infant and toddler formula and foods adversely affects breastfeeding patterns and rates. In fact, research demonstrates that later rates of breastfeeding exclusivity and duration decrease as level of exposure to formula advertising increase (Greiner & Latham, 1982). The influence of advertising is more intense when women's breastfeeding goals are not clearly defined; positive guidance and support for these decisions during the prenatal period is potentially highly influential (Howard, Weitzman, Lawrence, & Howard, 1994). Commercial advertisers are aware of this potential; formula advertisements and samples are available in 73% of Family Practice offices, 54% of OB/Gyn's offices, and 36% of Nurse Midwives' offices (Dusdieker, Dungy, & Losch, 2006). Further, new research indicates that prenatal women may be even more susceptible to being misled by formula marketing than women at other times in their reproductive lifecycle (Parry et al., 2013).

Text for Baby

Text4baby is a free mobile information service designed to provide pregnant women and moms of babies under one with information to help them care for their health and give their babies the best possible start in life. Text4baby reinforces messages about breastfeeding with information developed in collaboration with a number of medical, public health, and experts, including a breastfeeding committee, to ensure that content is medically accurate, communicates a positive and encouraging tone, provides guidance on topics and timing of critical breastfeeding messages, and assesses external feedback. Women can sign up by **texting BABY to 511411** (or BEBE in Spanish) to receive free messages timed to their due date or baby's date of birth. Those who enroll receive up to three messages a week, including this message sent in pregnancy: "Are you thinking about breastfeeding? Breast milk is the best food for babies. To learn more about breastfeeding, call 800-994-9662." This text4baby message is sent to moms of infants: "Back to work? At work, you have the right to pump milk to save for later. Breastfeeding helps you & your baby re-connect at the end of each work day." If you work with pregnant women and new moms, encourage women to sign up for critical health, safety, and breastfeeding information by becoming a text4baby partner and helping to spread the word. Visit www.text4baby.org for more information and access to all of the resources and materials.

"I got a few texts about breastfeeding and learned how much it can help my baby. I talked about it with my doctor and ended up breastfeeding and pumping for almost a year after she was born." — Text4baby mom, Chicago

---

Perinatal/Birth

Perinatal Health Service and Provider-Related Influences on Exclusive Breastfeeding

The policies, training, protocols, and practices of healthcare personnel at the site and time of birth are highly associated with establishment and duration of EBF.

Multiple studies demonstrate that exclusive breastfeeding initiation and duration rates increase when babies are born in baby-friendly hospitals (Biro, Sutherland, Yelland, Hardy, & Brown, 2011; Broadfoot, Britten, Tappin, & MacKenzie, 2005; Merten et al., 2005; Philipp, Malone, Cimo, & Merewood, 2003). Baby-Friendly Hospital Certification is granted when there is evaluated adherence to the Ten Steps to Successful Breastfeeding (see Table 3.1).

Table 3.1. Ten Steps to Successful Breastfeeding.

1	Have a written breastfeeding policy that is routinely communicated to all health-care staff.
2	Train all healthcare staff in skills necessary to implement this policy.
3	Inform all pregnant women about the benefits and management of breastfeeding.
4	Help mothers initiate breastfeeding within half an hour of birth.
5	Show mothers how to breastfeed, and how to maintain lactation, even if they should be separated from their infants.
6	Give newborn infants no food or drink other than breast milk, unless medically indicated.
7	Practice rooming-in - that is, allow mothers and infants to remain together - 24 hours a day.
8	Encourage breastfeeding on demand.
9	Give no artificial teats or pacifiers (also called dummies or soothers) to breast-feeding infants.
10	Foster the establishment of breastfeeding support groups and refer mothers to them on discharge from the hospital or clinic.

Source: WHO/UNICEF, 1989

Babies born in BFHI-certified facilities are 28% more likely to be exclusively breastfed when compared to babies born in hospitals in the process of becoming BFHI-certified or those who have made no efforts towards certification, and there is a doubling of average EBF duration from six to 12 weeks (Merten et al., 2005; Philipp et al., 2003). Increasing the number of Ten Steps that are in place in a hospital is associated with a dose response in achieving exclusive breastfeeding intentions (Declercq, Labbok, Sakala, & O'Hara, 2009). BFHI-certified maternity facilities where nurses received additional breastfeeding training beyond the basic course may experience even more significant increases in rates of EBF (Martens, 2000). However, only about 5% of maternity facilities in the U.S. are certified "Baby-Friendly" (Baby Friendly USA, 2012). Designations are on the rise since 1996 as shown in Figure 3.3. Globally, increases in the percent of hospitals certified have varied over time and by region (Figure 3.4; Labbok, 2012).

Figure 3.3. Increasing Number of BFHI Facilities in the USA.

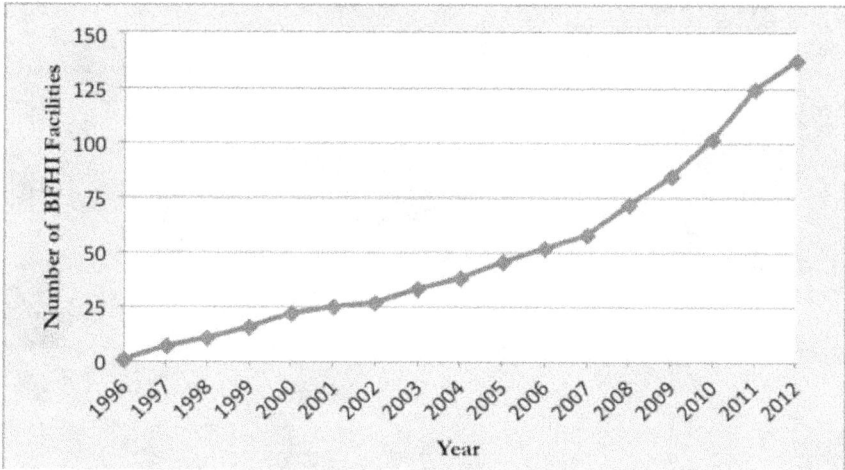

Source: Baby Friendly USA. Used with permission.

Figure 3.4 Percent of Hospitals Ever Designated "Baby-Friendly" Has Varied by Region and Over Time.

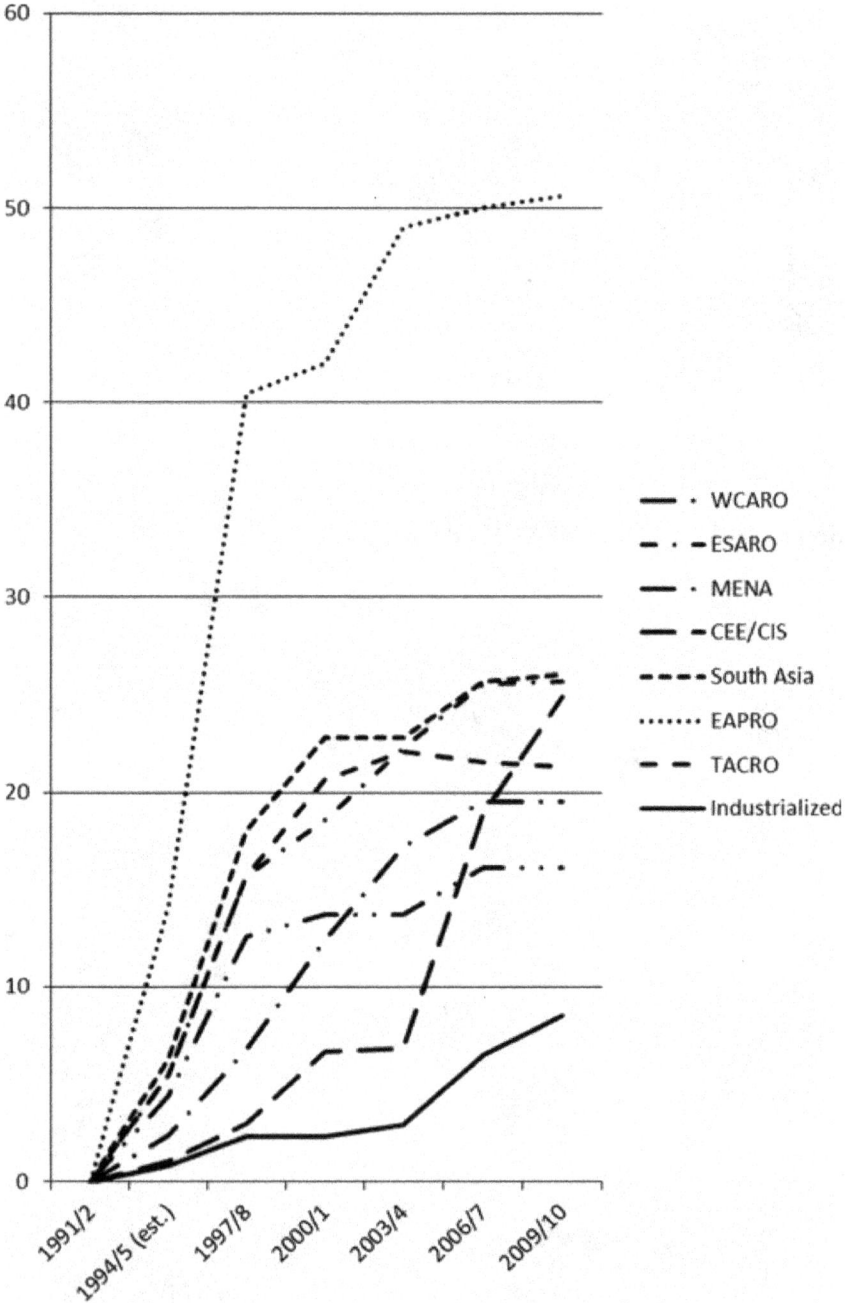

Regional abbreviations: WCARO – West and Central Africa (Regional Office); ESARO- East and Southern Africa (Regional Office); MENA – Middle East and North Africa; CEE/CIS – Central and Eastern Europe and Commonwealth of Independent States; EAPRO- East Asia and Pacific Rim (Regional Office); TACRO – The Americas and Caribbean (Regional Office) **Source:** Labbok M. 2012. Used with permission.

Rates of exclusive breastfeeding are associated with mode of delivery (Al-Sahab, Lanes, Feldman, & Tamim, 2010; Dewey, Nommsen-Rivers, Heinig, & Cohen, 2003; Rowe–Murray & Fisher, 2002; Semenic et al., 2008; Zanardo et al., 2010). Medical intervention during labor and delivery has risen drastically over the last 15 – 20 years, introducing multiple factors with potential influence on exclusive breastfeeding. For example, the rate of labor induction in the U.S. rose 143% in the last two decades – from 9.5% in 1990 to 23.1% in 2009 (Martin et al., 2006; Martin et al., 2011). Receiving anesthesia during labor and delivery, especially in the form of epidurals, is significantly associated with earlier cessation of EBF (Clifford, Campbell, Speechley, & Gorodzinsky, 2006; DiGirolamo, Grummer-Strawn, & Fein, 2008).

Physician attended deliveries may be associated with a higher rate of medical procedures. Cesarean section, in particular, is associated with lower rates of breastfeeding success. One study included only low-risk women and found that epidural anesthesia and oxytocin for induction and augmentation were used significantly more frequently in the physician-managed patients. Both of these interventions are associated with an increased rate of Cesarean section. This study found that nurse-midwife-managed patients had a significantly lower rate of Cesarean section (8.5% versus 12.9%; P < .005) and operative vaginal delivery (5.3% versus 17%, P = .0001) than the physician-managed patients (Davis, Riedmann, Sapiro, Minogue, & Kazer, 1994). In 2009, 98.9% of all births occurred in hospitals, 86.7% occurring with physicians attending (Martin et al., 2011). Midwives attended 7.4% of all hospital births in 2009 (Martin et al., 2011).

There is a risk of change in rates of breastfeeding if rates of invasive procedures, such as Cesarean section, continue to increase as shown in Figure 3.5. The rate of exclusive breastfeeding is significantly lower among mothers giving birth by Cesarean section as compared with mothers giving birth vaginally (Al-Sahab et al., 2010; Clifford et al., 2006; Ludvigsson & Ludvigsson, 2005; Semenic et al., 2008; Zanardo et al., 2010). While the rate of Cesarean deliveries declined between 1989 (22.8%) and 1996 (20.7%), it has risen steadily to 32.9% in 2009 (Martin et al., 2011). The increase in Cesarean births is also likely to affect the rates of exclusive breastfeeding. Delivery by Cesarean has been shown to significantly predict in-hospital formula supplementation (Biro et al., 2011). In fact, mothers giving birth vaginally are more than one and one half (1.5) times more likely to initiate exclusive breastfeeding (Pechlivani et al., 2005). This association may be due to the impact of the surgery and length of hospital stay, use of anesthesia, lack of physiologically complete labor, or a combination of these (and other potential) factors (Clifford et al., 2006; Rowe–Murray & Fisher, 2002; Simopoulos & Grave, 1984).

Figure 3.5. Increasing Rates of Cesarean Section in the USA.

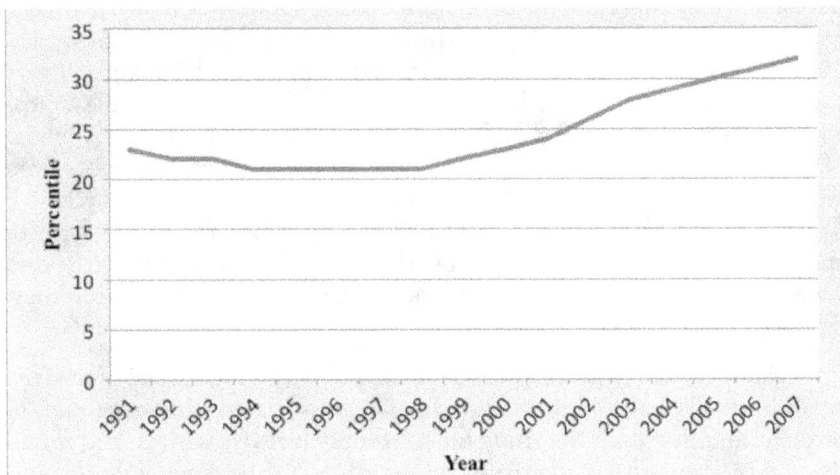

Data Source: CDC/NCHS, National Vital Statistics System.

Perinatal Social, Economic, and Political Influences on Exclusive Breastfeeding

No studies were found that addressed social, economic, or political influences on the impact birthing practices would have on exclusivity of breastfeeding, although there is a considerable literature on cultural and traditional birthing practices, birth attendants and length of labor, and possible associations with breastfeeding in general.

Perinatal Media and Marketing Influences on Exclusive Breastfeeding

No studies specific to this issue and time were identified.

Immediate Postpartum Period / Hospital Stay

The events of the immediate postpartum period are highly associated with initiation, duration, and exclusivity of breastfeeding. Ninety-nine percent of births in the U.S. occur in hospitals, where the average length of stay for uncomplicated vaginal delivery is 2.1 days, and an average of 1.2 days longer following Cesarean sections (Russo, Wier, & Steiner, 2006).

> ### Joint Commission "Speak Up Initiative"
>
> In March 2002, The Joint Commission, together with the Centers for Medicare and Medicaid Services, launched a national campaign to urge patients to take a role in preventing healthcare errors by becoming active, involved, and informed participants on the healthcare team. The program features brochures, posters, and buttons on a variety of patient safety topics.
>
> - Speak Up: What you need to know about breastfeeding in the hospital was added in August of 2011 and is available for download and distribution.
>
> http://www.jointcommission.org/speakup_breastfeeding/

Health Service and Provider-Related Influences on Exclusive Breastfeeding in the Immediate Postpartum Period

Lack of sufficient milk production in the early postpartum period may result from pre-existing conditions, such as maternal diabetes, obesity, blood transfusions, prolonged and/or complicated labor, etc. There are rare cases of low to no maternal milk production associated with conditions such as polycystic ovarian syndrome, breast reduction surgery, etc. (Chapman & Perez-Escamilla, 1999; Dewey et al., 2003). These conditions and situations can be addressed by the health system. For example, skilled providers and availability of banked donor human milk can be vital in adequately addressing such obstacles. There are also many factors with potential to disrupt the maternal-infant bond, including low birthweight infants (8.2% of births in 2009; Martin et al., 2011); severely ill infants; Cesarean births (32% of all births); and postpartum depression (following approximately 13% of births; Dennis & McQueen, 2009). However, these difficulties can be overcome, at least in part, by active support for the mother/baby relationship via hospital practices.

Research suggests that selected issues found in the Ten Steps can have a particularly strong impact on rates of EBF. DiGirolamo et al. (2008) found that women who experience fewer of the Ten Steps are more likely to terminate breastfeeding before six weeks. Similarly, Chalmers et al. (2009) suggest that insufficient adherence to several of the Ten Steps may be contributing to the shorter duration of exclusive breastfeeding. A study in Taiwan demonstrated that the more steps a woman reported receiving, the more likely she was exclusively breastfeeding at hospital discharge, one month, and three months postpartum, and delivering in a Baby-Friendly hospital increases the odds of a woman receiving each individual step (Chien, Tai, Chu, Ko, & Chiu, 2007).

Mothers and babies who room-in during their hospital stay have significantly higher rates of exclusive breastfeeding (Pechlivani et al., 2005), and couplets who initiate breastfeeding within one hour of birth have a longer duration of breastfeeding (DiGirolamo et al., 2008). Immediate skin-to-skin contact and early breastfeeding on-demand are proven to heavily influence EBF success because normal establishment of feeding and frequency of feeds correlate with establishment of sufficient milk supply (Kurinij & Shiono, 1991; Pechlivani et al., 2005), which in turn can decrease early complications that might occur due to milk stasis (lack of milk removal). Exclusive breastfeeding rates also appear to decline with early use of pacifiers (DiGirolamo et al., 2008; Howard et al., 2003; Kronborg & Væth, 2009; Scott, Binns, Oddy, & Graham, 2006), which is a common practice in hospitals (44%; Declercq, Sakala, Corry, & Applebaum, 2007).

Breastfed infants born in hospitals that are not accredited with BFHI designation are more likely to receive supplementation (Biro et al., 2011). There is strong evidence that the introduction of human milk substitutes without medical indication has deleterious effects on exclusive breastfeeding success (DiGirolamo et al., 2008; Donnelly, Snowden, Renfrew, & Woolridge, 2001; Frank, Wirtz, Sorenson, & Heeren, 1987; Howard et al., 1994; Petrova, Hegyi, & Mehta, 2007; Wright, Parkinson, & Scott, 2006). One study found that only 13% of infants who were supplemented in the hospital were fed substitutes for reasons that meet ABM indications for supplementing (Tender et al., 2009). Wright and colleagues found that regularly administering supplementary feeds leads to a ten-fold increase in the odds of women ceasing breastfeeding by hospital discharge (Wright et al., 2006). Commonly cited reasons for feeding infant formula in the hospital are "poor weight gain," "problems with the latch," or "mother needs rest" (Kurinij & Shiono, 1991; Taveras et al., 2004). In addition, unnecessary administration of these substitutes reinforces one of women's most commonly cited reasons for not exclusively breastfeeding: concerns about milk supply (Cohen, Brown, Rivera, & Dewey, 1999; Gatti, 2008). A systematic review of articles discussing perceived milk supply shows that many studies demonstrate a correlation between perceived insufficient milk supply and decreased EBF (Gatti, 2008). Women's perceptions that they are likely to fail are validated when hospital providers distribute discharge bags containing commercial infant formula (Parry et al., 2013); they often believe their providers are endorsing the product brand (Grummer-Strawn, 2006; Rosenberg, Eastham, Kasehagen, & Sandoval, 2008). In a recent study, racial/ethnic groups reported differing levels of in-hospital supplementation, with varying percentages continuing exclusive breastfeeding at one month postpartum (see Table 3.2; Petrova et al., 2007).

Table 3.2. Data Derived from New Jersey Study with Additional Calculations and Rounding.

Race/Ethnicity	Percent of each Race/ Ethnicity EBF in Hospital	Percent of each Race/ Ethnicity EBF at 1 month	Of those reporting EBF in hospital (Col. 2, n=157), EBF at 1 month	Of those reporting not EBF in hospital, (100%-Col. 2, n=150) EBF at 1 month
% (n)	% (n)	% (n)	% (n)	% (n)
White 54.1 (166)	54.2 (90)	34.9 (58)	55.6 (50)	10.5 (8)
Black 10.1 (31)	38.7 (12)	29.0 (9)	50.0 (6)	15.8 (3)
Asian 20.5 (63)	54.0 (34)	41.3 (26)	58.9 (20)	20.7 (6)
Hispanic 15.3 (47)	44.7 (21)	10.7 (5)	19.1 (4)	3.9 (1)
Total 100 (307)	**51.1 (157)**	**32.0 (98)**	**50.9 (80)**	**12.0 (18)**

Source: Petrova et al., 2007. Used with permission.

A recent study also underscores that influences on EBF vary by racial/ Ethnic grouping. The most influential predictors (P<0.001) were attitude for white mothers, subjective norm for African-American mothers, and perceived behavioral control for Latina mothers. Latent beliefs strongly associated with attitude in white mothers were 'bonding with the baby' and 'easy feeding.' Beliefs held by family members and the general public contributed to the subjective norm of African-American mothers. Perceived behavioral control in Latina mothers was highly correlated with 'pumping breast milk' (Bai, Wunderlich, & Fly, 2011).

Infants who require hospitalization after birth often have special nutrition needs. The barrier to breastfeeding caused by maternal/infant separation can be overcome by supporting the mother to express her own milk until the infant can breastfeed directly, or by use of donor human milk for the infant, wherever possible. One small study of infants in the NICU found that longer length of stay was the main determinant of cessation of maternal milk expression (Maia, Brandao, Roncalli, & Maranhao, 2011). Dr. Jane Morton attempted to overcome this barrier of continued milk expression: she found that hand expression combined with pump use yields a greater usable supply of colostrum and higher caloric milk among mothers of preterm infants (Morton et al., 2009; Morton et al., 2012). The implication of this finding is that pump expression in concert with hand expression may be additive in contributing to continued use of mother's milk and/or breastfeeding following NICU hospitalization. Further, a comprehensive intervention in the NICU significantly increased EBF rates on the infant's first day home after discharge from the NICU, and this effect was more pronounced for VLBW infants. The intervention was implemented over several years and included IBCLC consults, a mothers' pumping room, NICU staff breastfeeding education, parental pamphlet education, use of galactagogues where necessary, simultaneous (both breasts) pumping, and weekly breastfeeding meetings with mothers while their baby was hospitalized (Dall'Oglio et al., 2007). A systematic review of NICU breastfeeding interventions confirmed the effectiveness of the following interventions: skin-to-skin, lay support, simultaneous milk expression (pumping both breasts), staff training, BFHI implementation, and the cost-effectiveness of skilled support from trained staff (Renfrew et al., 2009).

Supporting Human Milk Banks through Mentorship
(Human Milk Banking Association of North America©
https://www.hmbana.org/establish-milk-bank)

Human Milk Banking Association of North America (HMBANA) facilitates the establishment of non-profit donor milk banks in North America in areas where they are needed. Their "Guidelines for the Establishment and Operation of a Donor Human Milk Bank" offers that if you are interested in establishing a human milk bank that you follow specific steps:

- Review *Best Practice for Expressing, Storing and Handling Human Milk in Hospitals, Homes and Child Care Settings* and complete a self-assessment (available on line) to ensure that you are able to consider going forward.

- If self-appraisal is accepted, HMBANA assigns a HMBANA mentor for up to two years.

- Upon the recommendation of your mentor, you may contact HMBANA Headquarters for the Developing Milk Bank application.

http://www.hmbana.org

Ongoing support, in the hospital and beyond, is associated with EBF success. The presence of knowledgeable breastfeeding social support in the early postpartum period, in addition to the Ten Steps, may be critical to increase EBF rates (Chapman et al., 2004; Verma et al., 1995). In fact, when support comes from lay advocates in private hospitals, there appears to be an even greater effect on EBF rates than on partial BF rates (Chung, Raman, Trikalinos, Lau, & Ip, 2008; Sikorski, Renfrew, Pindoria, & Wade, 2003; Truitt, Fraser, Grimes, Gallo, & Schulz, 2003). In retrospective analysis, mothers reported that if they had not had staff support, they would have been more likely to stop EBF earlier (Cohen et al., 1999). Thus, hospitals that do not ensure that there is social and staff support available may be presenting a significant constraint to EBF. A qualitative study of nurses, midwives, patients, and partners revealed that care providers did not have enough time to support maternal breastfeeding skills, further emphasizing a need for more readily available professional lactation support in postpartum settings (Gilmour, Hall, McIntyre, Gillies, & Harrison, 2009). Evidence suggests that when hospitals try to initiate the Ten Steps, they do better in training personnel and providing women with health education on breastfeeding than on those steps which require a change in clinical practice (Chien et al., 2007). Educating nurses on breastfeeding improves their confidence in practice (Watkins & Dodgson, 2010) and improves breastfeeding knowledge, attitudes, and practice intentions (Bernaix, Beaman, Schmidt, Harris, & Miller, 2010). The type of educational intervention most likely to be effective remains to be demonstrated (Spiby et al., 2009; Watkins & Dodgson, 2010).

A recent article estimated the number of Internationally Board Certified Lactation Consultants (LCs) full time equivalents (FTEs) needed for sufficient support in a tertiary care medical center (Mannel & Mannel, 2006). Table 3.3 presents the FTE ration of LCs needed, given that an effective lactation program should offer:

- Clinical Services: inpatient consults, outpatient consults, and telephone consults

- Education Services: staff/physician education (including LCs), student education (nursing, medical), and preceptorships

- Research: process improvement, product/ equipment trials, and clinical research

- Program Development/Administration: policies, procedures, documentation, staffing, personnel management, patient information, statistics/productivity, quality assurance, and hospital leadership

It is proposed that, rather than utilizing one "global" ratio for calculating staffing, the ratios in Table 3.3 allow hospital administrators to calculate IBCLC staffing based on the number of deliveries, breastfeeding rate, and extent of services desired.

Table 3.3. Ratios for Calculating the Numbers of Full Time Equivalent (FTE) Lactation Consultants Necessary in a Hospital Setting.

Service	FTE Ratio
Mother/baby coverage (inpatient)	1:783 breastfeeding couplets
Neonatal Intensive Care Unit (NICU) coverage (inpatient)	1:235 infant admissions
Post-discharge coverage	
- Mother/baby outpatients	1:1292 breastfeeding couplets
- Mother/baby telephone follow-up	1:3915 breastfeeding couplets
- NICU outpatients	1:818 breastfeeding infants
- NICU telephone follow-up	1:3915 breastfeeding infants
Education	0.1:1000 deliveries
Program development/administration	0.1:1000 deliveries
Research	0.1-0.2 FTE total

Source: Mannel & Mannel, 2006.

The Mary Rose Tully Training Initiative

The Mary Rose Tully Training Initiative (MRT-TI) was initiated and developed in 2009 by the Carolina Global Breastfeeding Institute in collaboration with the UNC Women's and Children's Hospital and the UNC Gillings School of Global Public Health. This IBLCE Pathway 2 program is unique in that it is:

- Developed as a regular course of study within an academic Health Sciences Center.

- Formed as a collaboration between the School of Public Health and the hospital.

- Open to graduate students as part of their on-site academic training.

The MRT-TI is one academic year and includes 120 hours of didactic training, for which students earn a total of six academic credits from the Gillings School of Global Public Health. Students also complete 300 hours of supervised clinical training at local medical training centers. The didactic and clinical components of the lactation program may be taken as part of a student's regular course of study within all graduate schools and undergraduate nursing programs. The course is entirely residential, supportive of the course philosophy of active and reflective learning. During each of their clinical experiences, students journal that experience, and then two students share formal case study presentations at each weekly didactic session.

Hormonal contraception in the immediate postpartum period is another important factor to consider when eliminating barriers to EBF at the healthcare level. It is a commonly reported practice to prescribe hormonal contraception during this period despite the possible risk of inhibiting the normal physiological onset of lactogenesis. The WHO advises against such practices (World Health Organization, 2009), while in the United States, the CDC classifies postpartum administration of progestin-only contraception methods as category 2 (advantages outweigh risks; Centers for Disease Control and Prevention, 2011b). Research on this issue is inconclusive (Chen, Reeves, Creinin, & Schwarz, 2011; Gurtcheff et al., 2011; Halderman & Nelson, 2002). However, a recent study calls into question the administration of progestin-containing contraceptives to women in the early postpartum period, pointing out the multiple methodological flaws of previous inconclusive research on the practice. In a RCT, the authors demonstrate that women receiving a progestin IUD immediately postpartum have a significantly shorter breastfeeding duration than those who received the hormonal IUD at six to eight weeks postpartum (Chen et al., 2011). Further data regarding postpartum contraception and exclusive breastfeeding are discussed in the time point Day 12 through Week Six.

Social, Economic and Political Influences on Exclusive Breastfeeding in the Immediate Postpartum Period

Family and friends can be influential in the success of breastfeeding and may encourage a mother to offer supplementation to her infant if she is experiencing difficulties getting breastfeeding started. A qualitative study offered a rich exploration of factors associated with early cessation of breastfeeding (Gilmour et al., 2009). Gilmour and colleagues found that new parents may be overwhelmed with information in the hospital at a time when they are extremely tired. This is further compounded by the constant distraction by visitors, phone calls, and the in-room television. For mothers who lack confidence or are uncomfortable with learning this new skill in the presence of others, the social environment of the hospital room discourages the establishment of successful breastfeeding.

Family and friends have a measurable influence on a woman's intention to breastfeed. As previously mentioned, a woman's intention to breastfeed is highly correlated with her initiation of breastfeeding in the hospital (Mistry et al., 2008), as well as exclusivity and duration (Bai et al., 2010; Dabritz et al., 2010). In addition, women who planned to breastfeed for four months or less are more likely to stop breastfeeding by four weeks than those who intended to breastfed for six months, according to analysis of several studies (Gilmour et al., 2009).

Marketing of Commercial Infant Formula: Influence on Exclusive Breastfeeding During the Immediate Postpartum Period

There is a strong inverse association between marketing of commercial feeding products in the immediate postpartum period and rates of exclusive breastfeeding (Dungy, Christensen-Szalanski, Losch, & Russell, 1992; Greiner & Latham, 1982; Rosenberg et al., 2008). This relationship was the basis for the acceptance of the WHO *International Code of Marketing of Breast-Milk Substitutes* (1981) articles that state substitutes for human milk should not be marketed in ways that interfere with breastfeeding (World Health Organization, 1981). The United States was the only nation to vote against adoption of the Code at that time (Rosenberg et al., 2008). The inverse relationship between advertising of formula and EBF rates is higher among women who are uncertain about their goals for breastfeeding as compared to women who are committed to exclusively breastfeeding before being exposed to formula advertising (Howard et al., 1994).

Some hospitals in the United States enter into agreements with formula companies wherein they receive discounted or free infant formula in exchange for distributing marketing materials to new mothers in the form of free hospital discharge bags (Baumslag & Michels, 1995) that contain free samples of formula, information on formula feeding, and discount coupons for future purchases of formula. Research demonstrates that women who receive these gift bags discontinue EBF earlier than those who do not receive the bags (Donnelly et al., 2001; Frank et al., 1987; Rosenberg et al., 2008). One study compared EBF rates among mothers who received traditional formula-filled discharge bags with mothers who received bags with a pump and no formula; women who received the pump and no formula exclusively breastfed approximately one and one half (1.5) times as long as women who received the free formula (4.18 weeks and 2.78 weeks, respectively; Baumslag & Michels, 1995). Another study found that women who did not receive discharge packs were more likely to be exclusively breastfeeding at three weeks postpartum (Rosenberg et al., 2008).

Interstate Collaborative

Due to lagging progress in Baby-Friendly Hospital designations, many states have developed programs to support hospital-level implementation of the Ten Steps to Successful Breastfeeding with varied success.

The Interstate Collaborative to Support Widespread Implementation of the Ten Steps to Successful Breastfeeding was launched in October 2011 by the Carolina Global Breastfeeding Institute, with support from AHRQ, to serve as a conduit for sharing among these active states.

This federally-funded collaborative is designed to:

- Support increased implementation of the Ten Steps to Successful Breastfeeding, a set of evidence-based hospital practices known to support optimal infant feeding.

- Define the issues and challenges associated with hospital-level implementation of the Ten Steps to Successful Breastfeeding.

- Develop a research agenda or strategy for further study of these problems.

- Share and summarize research findings and evidence-based information and tools with individuals and organizations in positions to use this information to improve outcomes and quality of Ten Step Implementation programs in the United States.

Participants in the Collaborative bring their valuable experiences to teach and learn together, and jointly develop a research agenda and quality improvement strategy that will best meet the needs of their state and others. The Collaborative is ongoing and expanding, and will soon be open to all states.

Days Three Through Twelve

Days three through 12 are of critical importance to exclusive breastfeeding success for two primary reasons:

- Mothers are just coming home and establishing routines with their new babies.

- Their milk supply is still being established (lactogenesis II-III).

Once home, women's contact with healthcare providers is decreased.

Health Service or Provider-Related Influences to Exclusive Breastfeeding in Days Three through Twelve

Professionally facilitated group counseling, lay counseling, and peer counseling in the first few weeks postpartum all have beneficial effects on EBF rates. The benefit increases as frequency of visits increase (Anderson et al., 2005). Morrow and colleagues compared three levels of counseling to see how frequency of counseling influenced rates of EBF. They found that duration and exclusivity increased as frequency of counseling sessions increased, with 67% of mothers practicing EBF in the six-visit group, 50% in the three-visit group, and only 12% in the group with no counseling (Morrow et al., 1999). Other research also demonstrates the effectiveness of early breastfeeding support in prolonging EBF (Hopkinson & Konefal Gallagher, 2009; Kronborg, Væth, Olsen, Iversen, & Harder, 2007; Kruske, Schmied, & Cook, 2007; Su et al., 2007).

It is in these early days when women express concerns regarding adequacy of weight gain, fear of milk insufficiency, and concerns over breastfeeding problems (Cohen et al., 1999; Dewey et al., 2003; Kronborg & Væth, 2009; Taveras et al., 2004). Women with concerns about breastfeeding problems in the first four weeks are nearly twice as likely to cease breastfeeding as mothers who do not report problems (Scott et al., 2006). Women are at highest risk of early cessation due to perceived insufficiency of milk during these weeks (Gatti, 2008). Women may turn to pediatricians for breastfeeding advice during this time, especially when they are the only healthcare providers with whom mothers are in contact (Dillaway & Douma, 2004). Screening and appropriate counseling are therefore appropriate and necessary (Kronborg & Væth, 2009; Scott et al., 2006). The duration of EBF is significantly associated with pediatrician counseling (Osis et al., 2004). However, pediatricians often lack the knowledge they need to effectively counsel mothers on breastfeeding problems and techniques (Dillaway & Douma, 2004; Yarmo & Malin, 2005). Further data regarding pediatrician breastfeeding education and counseling are discussed in time point Week Six to Week 12.

Due to the current lack of pediatric specialized training in breastfeeding (Osband, Altman, Patrick, & Edwards, 2011) and time constraints in pediatric visits, many have considered the strategy of employing IBCLCs within pediatric offices. Witt et al. introduced a lactation consultant visit for all healthy newborns between three to five days of life. They found this to be a promising solution. Since the feeding assessment was conducted by a lactation consultant, the pediatrician only needed to precept the visit, spending approximately five minutes in the patient room. The practice was able to reduce the mean age at which infants were seen by more than five days, and breastfeeding initiation and intensity rates improved (Witt, Smith, Mason, & Flocke, 2012).

Social, Economic, and Political Influences on Exclusive Breastfeeding in Days Three Through Twelve

As women leave the hospital and return home with their new babies, their social sphere changes; the frequency of healthcare interactions decreases and more intimate interactions with family and friends become more important (Ruchala & Halstead, 1994). The major sociopolitical influences in days three through 12 are therefore family support and mother-infant bonding. Planning for return to work is also an often-cited factor.

Successful exclusive breastfeeding often involves mother-child bonding, as well as family support, especially from the parenting partner (Cernadas, Noceda, Barrera, Martinez, & Garsd, 2003; Kronborg & Væth, 2004). Securing and continuing a strong bond between mother and infant is critical to the continuation of exclusive breastfeeding at this phase. Research demonstrates that optimal bonding in the mother-child dyad increases duration of EBF (Cernadas et al., 2003).

Exclusive breastfeeding is increased when the family, especially the father, has a supportive attitude (Osis et al., 2004; Scott et al., 2001). Survey respondents in one study reported that the negative attitude of the baby's father toward breastfeeding was the number one reason for the introduction of formula (Scott et al., 2001). In a qualitative study, fathers report that their self-efficacy is especially low if breastfeeding becomes difficult for their partner, and formula allows them to be more involved in feeding (Sherriff & Hall, 2011). Supportive fathers typically offer encouragement in the more difficult moments of breastfeeding–approval, admiration, and appreciation–and practical support in terms of the household balance of labor.

Paternal support may encourage maternal pride and confidence, which have demonstrated an increased duration of EBF (Kronborg & Væth, 2004). Blyth et al. measured mother's breastfeeding self-efficacy prenatally, at one week postpartum, and again at four months postpartum. Findings demonstrated that high breastfeeding self-efficacy was associated with breastfeeding initiation and exclusivity at one-week postpartum, whereas low self-efficacy was related to bottle feeding. New mothers with higher self-efficacy were significantly more likely to continue to breastfeed to four months postpartum, and to do so exclusively, than mothers with lower scores (Blyth et al., 2002).

Marketing of Commercial Infant Formula: Influence on Exclusive Breastfeeding From Day Three to Twelve

There is a little research on how commercial infant formula marketing approaches influence infant feeding decisions. A recent qualitative study explores women's perceptions of various forms of formula marketing (Parry et al., 2013) and concludes that women understand they will likely not succeed in their breastfeeding goals after viewing infant formula advertisements and receiving samples. This expectation of failure that sets in after being exposed to formula marketing at the direct-to-consumer and healthcare outlet levels facilitates the ease with which women choose to supplement or wean when a problem or challenge with breastfeeding is encountered, rather than seek out professional support from a lactation consultant.

Day Twelve through Week Six

Rates of exclusive breastfeeding continue to drop rapidly between day 12 and week six. Milk supply is established during this period. This time is also unique in that most women are consistently alone with their babies for the first time, as family and friends return to their daily routines. Fathers typically take vacation time or unpaid time off from work for one to two weeks, but then return to work (varying, of course, by occupation; Hörnell, Hofvander, & Kylberg, 2001). Thus, women use day 12 through week six to establish routines of parenting – most importantly, sleeping and infant feeding patterns.

Health Systems and Provider-Related Influences on Exclusive Breastfeeding from Day Twelve through Week Six

Women who have breastfeeding problems in the first four weeks postpartum are nearly twice as likely to discontinue exclusive breastfeeding prematurely (Scott et al., 2006). The most common reasons for cessation cited during the first month are related to lactation and perceived nutrition (Li, Fein, Chen, & Grummer-Strawn, 2008). Breastfed infants who do not receive pacifiers are more than three times as likely to be fully breastfeeding at six months, when compared to those who did not receive pacifiers (23.3% vs. 7.1%, respectively; Scott et al., 2006). Both breastfeeding problems and introduction of pacifiers are constraints to EBF that can be mediated by knowledgeable breastfeeding counselors, trained peers, or visiting nurses (Anderson et al., 2005; Chapman et al., 2004; Kronborg & Væth, 2009; Sikorski et al., 2003). Thus, continued healthcare interaction focusing on the mother is beneficial to increasing success rates of EBF during day 12 through week six.

This is also a time when family planning is often considered. Given that some hormonal methods have been shown to compromise milk supply, inclusion of EBF support in family planning counseling is essential. EBF can be actively encouraged by the inclusion of the LAM (Lactational Amenorrhea Method) as an option among family planning choices discussed.

Taylor and Cabral have shown that there is a strong inverse association between unwanted pregnancies and breastfeeding among white women living in the United States (Taylor & Cabral, 2002), but this does not confirm causation. In fact, breastfeeding *per se* is not a reliable form of family planning for the individual. However, we know that the risk of conception among exclusively breastfeeding women who breastfeed day and night approaches zero throughout the first six weeks postpartum (Perez et al., 1979; Gray et al., 1990; Labbok et al., 1997). This and other research has shown that we can identify those specific parameters of breastfeeding associated with the suppression of adequate ovulation, and hence associated with fertility suppression (Kennedy et al., 1988). The method of family planning based on these parameters, which derive from breastfeeding physiology, is known as the Lactational Amenorrhea Method

(LAM; Labbok et al., 1994). The pattern of frequent infant suckling at the breast, mediated by the mammary–hypothalamic–pituitary–ovarian axis and feedback, results in suppression of ovulation, delaying the return of menses in the postpartum period (Gray et al., 1990). LAM is 99.5% effective with perfect use, and 98% effective with typical use during the first six months (Labbok et al., 1997). LAM may provide additional motivation to practice optimal infant feeding after week six, but only if women are aware of its efficacy and how to use it. There are indications that most American women and most healthcare providers are not aware of LAM or the exact criteria for its use.

Social, Economic, and Political Influences on Exclusive Breastfeeding from Day Twelve through Week Six

There is strong evidence suggesting that significant proportions of the U.S. adult population have negative attitudes related to breastfeeding. Women's confidence and sense of personal empowerment is critical to continuation of exclusive breastfeeding in this time period (Brown & Lee, 2011; Gilmour et al., 2009; Kronborg & Væth, 2004; Li et al., 2008). Widespread lack of societal support for breastfeeding is likely to diminish women's sense of confidence in their infant feeding choices, and could potentially be a factor in the significant decline in EBF at this critical period. For example, 45% of American adults surveyed said that breastfeeding mothers had to give up too many lifestyle choices (Li et al., 2002). Thirty-one percent (31%) believed that one-year-olds should not be breastfed, and 27% considered breastfeeding in public to be embarrassing. The social stigma associated with public breastfeeding is likely to prohibit women from breastfeeding in public, making exclusive breastfeeding much more difficult. This belief was especially prominent among individuals younger than 30 and older than 65, those with lower income, and those with less education (Li et al., 2002). In this scenario, exclusively breastfeeding women either are subjected to public "embarrassment" for feeding their infants or are relegated to private spaces with limited personal contact. Therefore, Americans' perception of public BF as something to be embarrassed about presents a significant constraint to women trying to practice optimal infant feeding.

Brown and Lee describe interviews with women who succeeded in exclusively breastfeeding for six months, noting that the women were confident and determined in their decision to EBF for six months, which may have helped them overcome barriers that cause other women to supplement or wean. Interviewees displayed behaviors associated with positive deviance, whereby they continued EBF despite receiving criticism or being in the minority. The women also reported high levels of support from family and peers, many having a friend or relative who had also breastfed (Brown & Lee, 2011).

The Influence of Media and Marketing on Exclusive Breastfeeding from Day Twelve through Week Six

Mothers' confidence in the quantity and quality of milk is important. A mother is likely to stop breastfeeding if she doubts the adequacy of her milk to meet the needs of her infant, regardless of the age of the infant (Li et al., 2008). Many advertisements targeting new mothers highlight the added nutritional components of the formula and their supposed benefit to infant health. These kinds of marketing tactics by infant formula manufacturers serve to undermine a woman's confidence in the sufficiency of her own milk to provide optimal nutrition to her infant (Parry et al., 2013). The marketing of toddler formulas also reinforces this misconception that formula has something added that a child needs above and beyond human milk.

Week Six Through Week Twelve

Health Service and Provider-Related Influences on Exclusive Breastfeeding from Six through Twelve Weeks

As has been previously established in this paper, healthcare interactions beyond the immediate postpartum period typically focus on the infant. Therefore, pediatricians have an important role in EBF protection and promotion in this time period when they are usually the only healthcare provider with whom the mother and baby come into contact. Pediatricians can be instrumental in preventing early weaning by making efforts to support breastfeeding mothers (Geraghty, Riddle, & Shaikh, 2008). AWHONN recently published a second edition of evidence-based clinical practice guidelines for breastfeeding support through the first year. Herein, a literature-based case is made for breastfeeding counseling at each and every interaction between the provider and the patient, most of which are postpartum in pediatric offices (Association of Women's Health Obstetric and Neonatal Nurses, 2007).

Considering the importance of pediatric support of breastfeeding, it is extremely problematic that pediatricians are not properly educated in breastfeeding or its management. According to a recent national survey of pediatric program directors, residents are provided with a median total of nine hours of breastfeeding training over three years (Osband et al., 2011). As a comparison, Lactation Consultants certified by the International Board of Lactation Consultant Examiners receive 90 hours of coursework in human lactation and an additional 300-1000 hours of lactation-specific clinical practice (International Board of Lactation Consultant Examiners, 2011). With such inadequate training, it is not surprising that pediatricians lack the necessary knowledge and skills to support women by addressing common problems (Taveras et al., 2004). One study interviewed mothers about the breastfeeding support they received at their pediatrician's office and found that only two of the 75 interviewed reported receiving hands-on support or referrals. Only a quarter of the interviewees reported their pediatrician expressed verbal support for breastfeeding (Cross-Barnet, Augustyn, Gross, Resnik, & Paige, 2012). Feldman-Winter and colleagues compared a 1995 pediatrician survey about breastfeeding to the results of the same survey in 2004 to assess change in attitudes and knowledge in that decade. Only 37% of respondents reported teaching breastfeeding techniques more than five times in the previous year, despite a high level of reported confidence for the management of breastfeeding problems. The 2004 survey results showed that although pediatrician's overall knowledge about breastfeeding is improving, attitudes and opinions are becoming less favorable. Fewer respondents thought that the benefits of breastfeeding outweighed the risks and fewer believed that all women are able to be successful at breastfeeding (Feldman-Winter, Schanler, O'Connor, & Lawrence, 2008).

Residency Curriculum Improves Breastfeeding Care

Feldman-Winter, L., Barone, L., Milcarek, B., Hunter, K., Meek, J., Morton, J., Williams, T., Naylor, A., & Lawrence, R.A. *Pediatrics*. 2010 Aug; 126(2):289-97.

The AAP residency curriculum was developed in response to evidence that physicians can make a difference in the protection, promotion, and support of exclusive breastfeeding, yet most physicians do not acquire the necessary knowledge and skills to adopt this role. The curriculum is competency driven, and is applicable for all primary care specialties. In a study of residency programs in pediatrics, obstetrics/gynecology, and family medicine, the curriculum successfully improved knowledge, practice patterns, and confidence among residents trained compared to residents that were not exposed to the curriculum. Additionally, exclusive breastfeeding rates increased at both initiation and six months among mothers surveyed in programs that implemented the curriculum.

Social, Economic, and Political Influences on Exclusive Breastfeeding from Six through Twelve Weeks

Analysis of extensive data from the Infant Feeding Practices Survey II reveals that the reported reasons for cessation of breastfeeding vary according to age of the infant. Generally speaking, the authors found that psychosocial and pumping-related reasons begin to gain importance as reasons for cessation between one and two months postpartum. Examples of reasons commonly cited during this time period include, "Breastfeeding is too inconvenient," "I have too many other household duties," "Pumping no longer seems worth the effort," "I didn't want to pump at work," "I wanted someone else to feed my baby," "I wanted to leave my infant for several hours at a time," and "I did not want to breastfeed my baby in public" (Li et al., 2008). These reasons point to the critical importance of a support system for mothers for continuing to EBF, not only in the household, but also in the community and in the workplace.

A systematic review of breastfeeding interventions including 38 randomized controlled trials highlights the effectiveness of lay support for breastfeeding mothers. Interventions included system-level breastfeeding support, formal breastfeeding education, professional support, and lay support. The breastfeeding interventions taken overall significantly increased short and long-term EBF when compared to usual care. Interventions involving lay support significantly increased EBF by 65% in the short term (Chung et al., 2008).

Influence of Media and Marketing on Exclusive Breastfeeding From Six Through Twelve Weeks

No studies specific to this issue and time were identified.

Month Three Through Month Six

Months three through six are defined as a critical period in the continuation of exclusive breastfeeding because a significant proportion of women prematurely wean their babies during this time (DHHS Centers for Disease Control and Prevention, 2012). Two of the most important factors include the return to work and misperceptions regarding infants' nutritional needs (Li et al., 2007). Reasons of perceived infant self-weaning also gain importance beginning at month three (Li et al., 2008).

Health Service and Provider-Related Influences on Exclusive Breastfeeding From Months Three Through Six

There are many common misperceptions regarding breastfeeding in the U.S. adult population (Li et al., 2007). For example, 31% thought that babies should be fed cereal or baby food by age three months (Li et al., 2002). Further, a study in Philadelphia found that individuals did not consider water, juice, or baby foods to be solids or "other than breastfeeding" (K. Hoover, personal communication, July 15, 2007). Healthcare personnel and parents should be aware that introduction of solids and introduction of formula can have very different consequences for continuation of any or exclusive breastfeeding; introduction of any formula can have a greater negative impact on the continuation of intensive breastfeeding than the introduction of a solid (Hörnell, Hofvander, & Kylberg, 2001). Moreover, research shows that misperceptions have only gotten worse in the last decade, with the percentage of respondents who believed that "infant formula is as good as breastmilk" increasing from 14.3% in 1999 to 25.7% in 2003, and 28% in 2005 (Centers for Disease Control and Prevention, 2005). Such erroneous beliefs regarding the inadequacy of breastfeeding (and the adequacy of formula) may be partially responsible for the high rates of premature introduction of complementary foods and use of commercial infant formula (Parry et al., 2013).

The AAP states that introduction of complimentary feedings before six months generally does not increase total caloric intake or rate of growth, and only substitutes foods that lack the benefits of human milk (Eidelman et al.,

2012). The AAP published recommendations for exclusive breastfeeding to about six months of infant age in 1997 (Gartner et al., 1997), 2005 (Gartner et al., 2005) and again in 2012 (Feldman-Winter, 2012), each citing the latest research that reinforce the conclusion that breastfeeding and human milk are the normative standard for infant feeding and nutrition (Eidelman et al., 2012).

Business Case for Breastfeeding

The Business Case for Breastfeeding is a national initiative of the U.S. Department of Health and Human Services, Health Resources and Services Administration's Maternal and Child Health Bureau, with additional funding from the HHS Office on Women's Health. The comprehensive, multi-faceted project includes:

- A resource toolkit, *The Business Case for Breastfeeding*, designed for employers, human resource managers, employees, and others involved in supporting breastfeeding employees at work. The kit is available online at the Office on Women's Health at:

  www.womenshealth.gov/breastfeeding/government-in-action/business-case-for-breastfeeding/. Hard copies are available free at the HHS HRSA Distribution Center at: www.ask.hrsa.gov.

- Community-based training events held with State Breastfeeding Coalitions and their partners in 30 U.S. States and six cities serviced by Healthy Start agencies. More than 3,000 breastfeeding educators and advocates have been trained across the country using the curriculum, "Implementing *The Business Case for Breastfeeding* in Your Community."

In addition to the toolkit, the Office on Women's Health has expanded the project through national level outreach with business organizations and labor unions, development of companion resources for hospitals and universities, training for work life coordinators of the Office of Personnel Management, and a national Business Case for Breastfeeding Summit.

In 2012 OWH began an initiative to target employers of overtime-eligible workers. The initiative included partnering with national business groups and selected state breastfeeding coalitions to develop an online searchable resource site providing solutions for time and space accommodations for breastfeeding workers in more challenging job settings.

Sociopolitical Influences on Exclusive Breastfeeding in Months Three Through Six

Women's decisions concerning return to the workplace have considerable influence on their rates of breastfeeding (Dearden et al., 2002; Fein & Roe, 1998; Flores, Pasquel, Maulén, & Rivera, 2005; Hawkins, Griffiths, Dezateux, & Law, 2007). Women who intend to return to work will have lower initiation rates that are directly associated with the length of leave. The largest influence is among women who must return to work for financial reasons (Raju, 2006). Moreover, women in more routine jobs are considerably less likely to exclusively breastfeed their infants at one and four months as compared to women in higher managerial positions (Kelly & Watt, 2005).

The return to work is a critical constraint to EBF that typically occurs at three months postpartum. Nearly 80% of women return to work by four months postpartum (Killien, 2005). Studies show that returning to work before six months postpartum is associated with decreased exclusive breastfeeding (Al-Sahab et al., 2010; Balkam, Cadwell, & Fein, 2011). Mandated extended maternity leave increases the duration of EBF by more than one-half month, and increases the proportion of mother-child pairs attaining six months of EBF (Baker & Milligan, 2008). Women typically wean their babies soon after returning to work, especially when they have not secured adequate support (Hawkins et al., 2007; Li et al., 2005). Lack of workplace support (breastfeeding rooms, scheduled breaks for milk expression, flexibility for working from home, etc.) has demonstrated especially deleterious effects on EBF (Balkam et al., 2011; Dearden et al., 2002; Fein, Mandal, & Roe, 2008; Hawkins et al., 2007). The work environments of people with higher socioeconomic status tend to be more supportive of breastfeeding (Fein & Roe, 1998). This fact alone could explain the difference in the rates of EBF occurring at three months in comparison to birth or one month (DHHS Centers for Disease Control and Prevention, 2012; see Table 1.1).

One study explores mothers' strategies who worked and breastfed; it examines intensity and duration of breastfeeding, as well as percentage of feedings from the breast (Fein et al., 2008). Upon the mother returning to work, the percentage of the infant's feeds that were human milk declined dramatically. Compared with directly feeding the infant from the breast during the workday, the strategy of pumping only was associated with 7.1 weeks shorter duration of breastfeeding. The authors advocate for more workplace support that encourages feedings at the breast, such as on-site childcare, telecommuting, and breaks where mother leaves to go feed or the infant is brought to her for feeding.

As women return to work outside of the home, they commonly entrust their babies to formal daycare providers or other caretakers who may or may not be related. The exclusively breastfed infant ideally has access to his or her mother for regular feedings. However, other caregivers can administer mothers' milk when appropriate storage and preparation amenities exist. Research suggests that daycare providers are not well informed in regards to supporting exclusive breastfeeding in these ways (Li et al., 2005). A recent study compared state and regional variation in infant feeding regulations for childcare facilities, and compared these regulations to national standards. The authors found that many states lacked infant feeding regulations at all (Benjamin et al., 2009). Moreover, Raju and colleagues found that formal daycares are typically so isolated from the workplace that women are restricted from visiting during the day to feed their infants (Raju, 2006).

Global – Grassroots Partnerships

Global non-governmental organizations (NGOs) and their national affiliates have done much to inspire, educate, and empower women and families, creating the energy for individuals, communities, and governments to make changes. Examples of this concept of global-grassroots collaboration include:

- La Leche League International, founded by a few breastfeeding moms in the Chicago area, became an international focus for mother-to-mother support.

- World Alliance for Breastfeeding Action (WABA) globally supports and promotes World Breastfeeding Week on the anniversary of the *Innocenti Declaration*, the first week in August. While many countries have switched the celebration to October, the global theme is acted upon at the community level. WABA has regional partners and an internationally representative Board.

- International Baby Food Action Network, which developed from multiple national partnerships, keeps individuals and policy makers alike aware of violations of the Code of Marketing of Breast-milk Substitutes by multinational corporations, addressing the risks of some public-private partnerships through on-going global grassroots coordination and collaborations.

The Influence of Media and Marketing on Exclusive Breastfeeding Between Three and Six Months

No studies specific to this issue and time were identified.

GAPS

There were many areas that emerged from this exploration where it was clear that additional research and study is needed. Table 3.4 presents a summary of the many areas meriting further exploration, so that they may best be translated into interventions and action approaches.

Table 3.4: Areas Where Additional Exploration Would Support Improved Translation

Health System or Provider-Related Research
• Effective pre- and inter-conceptional EBF counseling efforts
• Effective models for promoting EBF during prenatal care visits
• Full availability of banked donor human milk
• Confirmation of the optimal IBCLC: patient ratio
• Association between co-sleeping with mother and duration of exclusive breastfeeding
• Overall health and survival rates with maternal co-sleeping
• Identification of the most effective form of breastfeeding education for different types of healthcare providers and identifying which providers to train for highest impact on EBF
• Best interventions to appropriately improve cultural competency of providers related to EBF
• Impact of cultural competency of providers on EBF support
Social, Economic, and Political Research
• Comprehensive understanding of the potential for and economic implications of paid maternity leave in the U.S.
• Effective strategies for improving attitudes among the public at large
• Based on how best to improve attitudes, how best to increase awareness regarding EBF
• Effective interventions for empowering women to EBF in the U.S. social context
• Optimal mechanisms for improving fathers' and other familial attitudes regarding BF and EBF
• Factors that occur during six to 12 weeks postpartum that have the greatest impact on continuation of EBF
Media and Marketing of Commercial Infant Formula
• Impact of formula advertising at the various critical time periods and in various professional medical practices/offices
• Impact of exposure to marketing and media presentation of EBF over time
• Impact of media and marketing to mothers and families before and during pregnancy on EBF
• Impact of media and marketing to mothers and families in the postpartum period after hospital discharge on EBF

Chapter 4.
Translating the Findings

Suggestions for Innovative Implementation to Advance Exclusive Breastfeeding

This book reviews research and evaluation findings on the obstacles and opportunities related to exclusive breastfeeding, examining 1) health systems and providers, 2) social, economic, and political forces, and 3) marketing of human milk substitutes. Each of these is explored at eight critical stages in the decision-making and practice of exclusive breastfeeding. Exploration of such wide-ranging evidence, translation of evidence of varied quality, analytic approach and purpose, and creation of recommendations for implementation are always limited in some manner due to innate complexity of these issues themselves, as well as due to the fact that those who translate and implement bring their own experiences and biases to this exercise. It is important to consider these difficulties when extrapolating recommendations from these findings. Specifically, for translating the findings presented into suggestions and recommendations for innovative implementation, we invite the reader to consider that:

- The number of studies that address exclusive breastfeeding specifically is limited in the U.S. due to low levels of exclusivity and concomitant difficulties in identifying study participants.

- Many of the time periods and areas of interest, *per se*, have not been studied. Further, when intervention and outcomes are temporally separated, or when the intervention is diffuse, larger numbers and longer-term data gathering would be needed to assess impact. For example, researchers exploring the impact of images in the media observed during pre-conception on EBF that occurs many months later may perceive too many possible confounders and too much complexity for conventional research.

- The definitions of breastfeeding and exclusive breastfeeding used in the research vary, making it difficult to assess comparability between studies.

- Some of the available studies are of less than optimal design, possibly due to difficulties in carrying out research on long-term behavior and on later impact of behaviors and/or interventions.

Summary of the Obstacles and Facilitators Identified That May Lend Themselves to Translation into Actions to Increase Exclusive Breastfeeding

Healthcare Systems and Providers

Obstacles

- Limited provider awareness, knowledge, clinical skills, and social support practices for EBF, and limited self-awareness

- Excessive use of medical interventions during labor and delivery

- Insufficient attention to immediate skin-to-skin at birth and evidence-based breastfeeding support practices, such as safe co-sleeping

- Poor understanding that optimal infant feeding includes exclusive breastfeeding at the breast from birth

- Lack of adequate breastfeeding support in NICUs

- Lack of awareness of, access to, and use of donor human milk

Facilitators

- Implementation of the Ten Steps to Successful Breastfeeding and/or designation processes at the state level or the Baby-friendly Hospital Initiative

- Increase in the number and availability of International Board Certified Lactation Consultants and others with peer counseling or other brief trainings

- The AHRQ systematic review and meta-analysis (Ip et al., 2007)

Social, Economic, and Political factors

Obstacles

- Limited community, political, legislative, and regulatory awareness of the public health impact and concomitant limited attention to action

- Misperceptions and fears due to lack of societal awareness and support

- Lack of adequate lay support opportunities for breastfeeding mothers

- Limited third party payment for sufficient support

- Rarity of public health programming in support of EBF outside of WIC, and limitations within WIC

- Lack of paid maternity leave/brevity of any leave

- Minimal and variable workplace support for maintenance of exclusive breastfeeding

Facilitators

- The Healthy People decade goals include exclusive breastfeeding
- The *Surgeon General's Call to Action*
- Increasing availability of unbiased data on exclusive breastfeeding rates across the country and at the state and local levels
- The Patient Protection and Affordable Care Act

Media and Marketing

Obstacles

- Aggressive marketing of formula (samples, gifts, coupons) to mothers through hospitals and clinicians' offices
- Public misperceptions secondary to aggressive marketing to the public
- Lack of media representation in television and cinema of exclusive breastfeeding as normative behavior

Facilitators

- Increased positive and negative attention to breastfeeding in media
- Increased normalization of breastfeeding, at least in the immediate postpartum period, in television series

Translation into Programmatic Interventions

The majority of interventions designed to increase breastfeeding, in general, would also have a positive impact on exclusive breastfeeding. Therefore, the recommendations presented below select, where possible, and highlight those interventions that are more specific to enhancing exclusive breastfeeding *per se*, based on this review of the literature. Further, the following suggested actions are encouraged as part of a program of active multidisciplinary and multi-sectoral coordination and support. Those that demand little resource allocation may be more readily selected for immediate action. For those interventions that demand considerable resources, it may be necessary to develop a cost savings statement to use in discussion and arguments to support organizational, policy, or political change.

Table 4.1. Potential Areas Identified for Intervention: Recommendations for Action

	Healthcare and Provider	Socioeconomic and Political	Media and Marketing
Pre-/ Interconception	Include EBF planning in all patient/provider interactions. Increase access to contraception.	Promote women's empowerment and self-efficacy.	Incorporate BF education into schools to reduce potential impact of breastmilk substitute advertising.
Prenatal	Include EBF discussion in prenatal care visits, including recommendation of attendance in prenatal BF class. Ensure that breastfeeding-related prenatal care examination skills are in curricula. Ensure that breastfeeding-related PNC examination skills and explanation of need are in clinical guidance provided by professional groups to members. Provide appropriate nutrition and physical activity guidance to pregnant women. Increase access to prenatal care. Increase providers' cultural competency regarding EBF. Increase access to home visits by health professionals and peer educators. Increase access to prenatal breastfeeding education (classes). Implement and adhere to the Ten Steps/ BFHI in all maternity care facilities.	Improve social support for a women's prenatal intention to breastfeed her infant.	Discontinue practice of distributing infant formula samples and advertisements direct to consumers.

Labor and Birth	Provide support for maternal self-efficacy.	Develop community advocacy and demand for decreasing practices that are not medically indicated and for increased support for humane treatment of mother and baby.	Follow Code of Marketing articles on commercial formula provision in the hospital.
	Decrease interventions that are not medically indicated.		
	Encourage doula or similar companion.		
	Facilitate immediate postpartum skin-to-skin contact and support for breastfeeding initiation within the first hour after birth.		
	Decrease elective Cesarean births.		
	Train anesthesiologists to adhere to the ABM clinical protocol for anesthesia for the breastfeeding mother.		
	Implement and adhere to the Ten Steps/BFHI in all maternity care facilities.		

Birth to Three Days Postpartum	Increase ratio of on-site LC or other skills-trained healthcare personnel to number of births.	Address maternal and paternal expectations, especially if delivery varies from that expected.	Eliminate free or subsidized supplies to hospital or marketing in the form of take-home products or samples.
	Implement and adhere to the Ten Steps/BFHI in all maternity care facilities.	Discourage excessive social distraction until breastfeeding is well established.	
	Improve clinical use of family planning options appropriate to this period.	Increase planning for overcoming the potential obstacle of return to workplace.	
	Decrease rates of in-facility, non-clinically indicated supplementation with water, formula, or any other non-human milk substance.	Promote the understanding that any EBF is better than no EBF is an essential message for establishment of EBF.	
	Provide analgesia and anesthesia appropriate for the breastfeeding mother.		
	Discourage pacifier use by all breastfeeding families.		
	Increase support for EBF in the NICU setting.		
	Educate healthcare professionals about post-partum care practices that hinder exclusive breastfeeding.		
	Encourage feeding on-demand.		
	Counsel women with evidence-based anticipatory guidance, especially regarding lactogenesis, milk supply, and comfort.		
	Observe and correct (if necessary) milk transfer prior to discharge.		

Three Days to 12 Days Postpartum	Increase access to IBCLCs beyond the hospital stay.	Create a norm wherein this period of time is primarily for mother/infant mutual learning, rather than a time for significant social interaction and "baby viewing."	Eliminate free or subsidized supplies to hospital or marketing in the form of take-home products or samples.
	Provide skills and counseling training for pediatricians to address maternal expectations and common early BF problems.	Increase societal commitment to exclusivity.	
	Increase availability of BF counseling by nurses or peers.	Promote EBF among fathers and other family members.	
	Discourage pacifier use.		
12 Days – 42 Days	Include EBF support in family planning method selection.	Decrease societal stigma of BF.	Counter formula advertising with public health messages regarding breast milk's incomparability / superiority.
	Include LAM among choices.	Educate regarding benefits of BF and risks of supplementation.	Eliminate free or subsidized supplies to hospital or marketing in the form of take-home products or samples.
	Address maternal issues related to guilt/ shame, frustration, fear, exhaustion, etc.	Create safe, public spaces for BF.	
	Increase prevalence of breastfeeding support groups in healthcare facilities.	Expand family leave benefits to cover all workers and extend benefits to at least six weeks.	
	Increase availability of BF counseling by nurses or peers.		
Six Weeks – 12 Weeks	Increase support from nurses and peer support in clinical and home settings.	Establish and/or increase paid maternity leave where possible.	Discontinue practice of distributing infant formula samples and advertisements direct to consumers.

Three Months - Six Months	Train pediatricians in supporting optimal infant feeding as per the most recent AAP recommendations.	Increase compatibility of work and EBF by instituting mothers' rooms, scheduled breaks for milk expression, in-house daycares, and increasing flexibility to work from home.	Discontinue practice of distributing infant formula samples and advertisements direct to consumers.
	Increase availability of BF counseling by nurses or peers.	Educate daycare workers regarding optimal infant feeding and skills for feeding human milk.	
	Increase access to breast pumps for mothers who must be separated from their breastfeeding children.	Promote partnerships between employers and nearby daycare facilities.	

Suggested Innovations and Interventions

In addition to the evidence-based recommendations elucidated above, the authors offer the following additional recommendations for use in facilitating the continued achievement of EBF. Based on knowledge from reviewing the literature and experience from collaborating with other breastfeeding professionals over many years, these additional insights may be considered as commentary on how many of the aforementioned recommendations for action may be implemented. In order for successful implementation of EBF-facilitating strategies to occur, prominent entities, such as federal and state governments, must provide continued support. These insights are therefore presented in such a way that suggests how governments and others in position of influence can use their offices to support breastfeeding.

Health Service and Provider-Related

1. Develop curricula for all healthcare workers that include lactational support, addressing delays in lactogenesis, and counseling skills, appropriate use of banked donor milk, and NICU support for EBF, as well as introduction of appropriate and evidence-based family planning during breastfeeding, while continuing efforts to implement breastfeeding-friendly hospital practices. Additionally, implement teaching of the AAP breastfeeding curriculum in all residency programs.

This recommendation could be articulated by government public health entities and presented to medical boards, hospital accreditation groups, and professional organizations for action.

2. Expand and revise third party payment to cover all aspects of breastfeeding support, and increase reimbursement of and access to professional lactation

consultant services (IBCLCs).

Private or government entities can work with major third party payers to develop cost savings models for coding and increased compensation for lactation support, including direct services and anticipatory counseling. These models would be made available to the public and other insurance entities for consideration.

Social, Economic, and Political

Socioeconomic

3. Reduce the economic challenges to EBF through increased support for paid maternity leave and workplace breastfeeding protection.

Expand support for paid maternity leave such that citizens of all nations enjoy this right. Countries without paid leave can look to developed countries with successful models in place for guidance. Additionally, governments can enforce regulations that protect breastfeeding break time and access to appropriate locations to breastfeed in the workplace.

4. Initiate social marketing for demand creation (i.e., creating social and societal demand for protection, promotion, and support of breastfeeding) for all recommendations in support of EBF, including improved health services, social and legislative support, and media and marketing improvements.

Federal, state, and private donor seed funding is encouraged to support non-governmental organizations (NGOs) and other community-oriented activity in this area.

5. Develop community social marketing approaches for EBF based on formative research for sub-populations, including a) addressing inequities in early access to quality care, b) demanding creation for reimbursement from third-party payers, c) emphasizing maternal self-efficacy, d) supporting mother/baby care together to reduce total number of appointments, and e) overcoming social and economic obstacles to EBF.

The federal government can encourage formative and translational research to provide the framework for targeted campaigns to address the specific social factors that create obstacles to EBF in different sub-populations. Federal, state, and private donor seed funding is encouraged to support NGO and other community-oriented activity in this area.

6. Implement the use of breastfeeding curriculum for childcare centers to ensure supportive staff, policies, and practices for all families.

Nationally funded campaigns to fight childhood obesity can include actions to support EBF in childcare facilities.

Political

7. Promulgate Federal/State legislation regarding aggressive marketing (i.e., legislate the Code of Marketing), legality of breastfeeding wherever mothers can be, and tax incentives for breastfeeding-friendly childcare centers and for employers who provide maternity leave, onsite childcare, and supportive accommodations.

This legislative action would depend on sufficient evidence-based research, demand creation, development and sponsorship of the pieces of legislation, and sufficient political will to pass them. Other legislation and tax-incentives can be implemented as needs arise.

8. Establish monitoring and regulation where legislation exists: third-party coverage, medical facility adherence to Ten Steps, WIC.

Government entities can create regulations based on existing and future health legislation and government position statements, such as GAO reports.

Media and Marketing

9. Continue to support the elimination of the distribution of free formula samples and coupons to the public, with special attention to impact such activities at healthcare outlets and marketing at points of sale.

While this may occur as a result of corporate action and/or public activism, appropriate government legislation will ensure attention to this issue.

10. Encourage or mandate regulation/self-regulation and monitoring by commercial formula manufacturers.

Although industry is cautious to avoid collusion, this issue could be framed as corporate social responsibility. The Pharmaceutical Research and Manufacturers of America (PhRMA) Code on Interactions with Healthcare Professionals (Pharmaceutical Research and Manufacturers of America, 2012) is an example of self-regulation by industry.

11. Encourage or mandate self-regulation and monitoring by multi-media organizations and major broadcasting companies.

Advertising of alcoholic beverages and tobacco products are currently self-regulated by most major broadcasting companies according to guidelines promulgated by authoritative organizations and/or government. Commercial infant formula advertising should be similarly regulated.

12. Develop a series of Public Service Announcements (PSAs).

Following the success of the OWH breastfeeding media campaign (DHHS Office on Women's Health, 2012), despite the compromises that occurred, it is reasonable to encourage broader use of public service announcements and other media outlets to encourage EBF. Such encouragement may come from associations and federal, state, and local governments. The Ad Council can be called upon to develop PSAs that specifically include self-efficacy, how to overcome obstacles to EBF, as well as importance of social/family support.

Chapter 5. The *Surgeon General's Call to Action to Support Breastfeeding*

We have identified the issue of exclusive breastfeeding, explored the literature and current activities, and presented and translated the findings into potential areas for action. Now let us look at how the EBF recommendations might complement and offer expansion of the considerations currently offered for action in the United States by the *Surgeon General's Call to Action to Support Breastfeeding*, which lays out seven action areas and twenty specific actions. Note: The table below omits comparison on Action Areas 17-20: Actions for Research and Surveillance.

Table 5.1. EBF Recommendations Include and Occasionally Go Beyond Current Breastfeeding Guidance

Surgeon General's Call to Action to Support Breastfeeding: Action Areas and Implementation Strategies	This review confirms recommendations for actions to support breastfeeding and/ or suggests additional actions to support Exclusive Breastfeeding, including to:
Actions for Mothers and Their Families:	
1. Give mothers the support they need to breastfeed their babies. Implementation Strategies: a) Help pregnant women to learn about the importance of breastfeeding for their babies and themselves. b) Teach mothers to breastfeed. c) Encourage mothers to talk to their maternity care providers about plans to BF. d) Support mothers to have time and flexibility to breastfeed. e) Encourage mothers to ask for help with breastfeeding when needed.	- Promote women's empowerment and maternal self-efficacy. - Address maternal issues related to guilt/ shame, frustration, fear, exhaustion, etc. - Increase planning for the potential obstacle of returning to work, with understanding that any EBF is better than no EBF as an essential message. - Increase access to breast pumps for mothers who must be separated from their children. - Create safe, public spaces for BF. - Improve social support for prenatal intentions to breastfeed. - Educate regarding the benefits of EBF and risks of supplementation.
2. Develop programs to educate fathers and grandmothers about breastfeeding. Implementation Strategies: a) Launch or establish campaigns for breastfeeding education that target a mother's primary support network, including fathers and grandmothers. b) Offer classes on breastfeeding that are convenient for family members to attend.	- Increase societal commitment to exclusivity. - Decrease societal stigma of breastfeeding. - Promote EBF among fathers and other family members.

Actions for Communities:	
3. Strengthen programs that provide mother-to-mother support and peer counseling. Implementation Strategies: a) Create and maintain a sustainable infrastructure for mother-to-mother support groups and care for peer counseling programs in hospital and community healthcare settings. b) Establish peer counseling as a core service available to all women in WIC.	- Increase availability of breastfeeding counseling by nurses or peers and allow access to home visits by health professionals and peer educators.
4. Use community-based organizations to promote and support breastfeeding. Implementation Strategies: a) Support and fund small nonprofit organizations that promote breastfeeding in communities of color. b) Integrate education and support for breastfeeding into public health programs that serve new families. c) Ensure around-the-clock access to resources that provide assistance with breastfeeding.	- Develop community advocacy and demand for decreasing maternity care practices that are not medically indicated. - Initiate social marketing for demand creation for all recommendations in support of EBF; federal, state, and private donor seed funding is encouraged to support NGOs and other community-oriented activity in this area.
5. Create a national campaign to promote breastfeeding. Implementation Strategies: a) Develop and implement a national public health campaign on breastfeeding that relies heavily on social marketing. b) Use a variety of media venues to reach young women and their families.	-Incorporate breastfeeding education into schools to reduce potential impact of breastmilk substitute advertising. - Counter formula advertising with public health messages re: breastmilk's superiority. - Develop a series of PSAs with the Ad Council specifically targeting how to overcome the obstacles to EBF, as well as the importance of maternal self-efficacy and social/family support. - Develop community social marketing approaches for EBF based on formative research.

6. Ensure that the marketing of infant formula is conducted in a way that minimizes its negative impacts on exclusive breastfeeding. Implementation Strategies: a) Hold marketers of infant formula accountable for complying with the Code. b) Take steps to ensure that claims about formula are truthful and not misleading. c) Ensure that healthcare clinicians do not serve as advertisers for infant formula.	- Discontinue practice of distributing infant formula samples and advertisements direct to consumers. - Follow the principles set forth in the Code of Marketing. - Legislate the Code of Marketing, legality of breastfeeding wherever mothers can be. - Encourage self-regulation and monitoring by multi-media organizations, major broadcasting companies, AND commercial infant formula manufacturers.
Actions for Health Care:	
7. Ensure that maternity care practices around the United States are fully supportive of breastfeeding. Implementation Strategies: a) Accelerate implementation of the Baby-Friendly Hospital Initiative. b) Establish transparent, accountable public reporting of maternity care practices in the U.S. c) Establish a new advanced certification program for perinatal patient care. d) Establish systems to control the distribution of infant formula in hospitals and ambulatory care facilities.	-Eliminate free or subsidized supplies to hospital or marketing in the form of take-home products or samples. - Implement and adhere to the Ten Steps/BFHI in all maternity care facilities. -Decrease elective Cesarean births and interventions that are not medically indicated; provide anesthesia appropriate to breastfeeding; encourage use of a Doula during labor. - Improve clinical use of family planning options appropriate to this period; include LAM among choices. - Discourage excessive social distraction until breastfeeding is well established.
8. Develop systems to guarantee continuity of skilled support for lactation between hospitals and healthcare settings in the community. Implementation Strategies: a) Create comprehensive statewide networks for home-or clinic-based follow-up to be provided to every newborn in the state. b) Establish partnerships for integrated and continuous follow-up care after discharge from the hospital. c) Establish and implement policies and programs to ensure that participants in WIC have services in place before discharge from the hospital.	- Observe and correct (if necessary) milk transfer prior to discharge. - Increase access to IBCLCs beyond the hospital stay. - Increase prevalence of breastfeeding support groups in healthcare facilities. - Increase availability of breastfeeding counseling by nurses or peers, and allow access to home visits by health professionals and peer educators.

9. Provide education and training in breastfeeding for all health professionals who care for women and children. Implementation Strategies: a) Improve the breastfeeding content in undergraduate and graduate education and training for health professionals. b) Establish and incorporate minimum requirements for competency in lactation care into health professional credentialing, licensing, and certification processes. c) Increase opportunities for continuing education on the management of lactation to ensure the maintenance of minimum competencies and skills.	- Develop curricula for all healthcare workers appropriate to EBF support. -Ensure breastfeeding-related examination skills are in curricula for preconception, prenatal and postpartum care, including addressing maternal expectations and common early breastfeeding problems. - Increase providers' cultural competency regarding EBF. - Train pediatricians in supporting EBF as per the most recent AAP guidelines. - Train anesthesiologists to adhere to the ABM clinical protocol for anesthesia for the breastfeeding mother.
10. Include basic support for breastfeeding as a standard of care for midwives, obstetricians, family physicians, nurse practitioners, and pediatricians. Implementation Strategies: a) Define standards for clinical practice that will ensure continuity of care for pregnant women and mother-baby pairs in the first four weeks of life. b) Conduct analyses and disseminate their findings on the comparative effectiveness of different models for integrating skilled lactation support into settings where midwives, obstetricians, family physicians, nurse practitioners, and pediatricians practice.	- Include discussion of EBF in all patient/provider interactions, including preconception planning and recommendation of prenatal breastfeeding class attendance. - Counsel women with evidence-based anticipatory guidance, especially regarding lactogenesis, milk supply, and comfort.
11. Ensure access to services provided by International Board Certified Lactation Consultants. Implementation Strategies: a) Include support for lactation as an essential medical service for pregnant women, breastfeeding mothers, and children. b) Provide reimbursement for IBCLCs independent of their having other professional certification or licensure. c) Work to increase the number of racial and ethnic minority IBCLCs to better mirror the U.S. population.	- Increase the ratio of onsite IBCLCs to number of births. - Increase access to IBCLCs beyond the hospital stay. - Expand and revise third party payment to cover all aspects of breastfeeding support. - Increase reimbursement of and access to IBCLC services.

12. Identify and address obstacles to greater availability of safe banked donor milk for fragile infants.	- Increase support for EBF in the NICU setting. - Include appropriate use of banked donor milk and NICU support for EBF in curricula for care providers.
Implementation Strategies:	
a) Conduct a systematic review of the current evidence on the safety and efficacy of donor human milk.	
b) Establish evidence-based clinical guidelines for the use of banked donor milk.	
c) Convene a study on federal regulation and support of donor milk banks.	
Actions for Employment:	
13. Work toward establishing paid maternity leave for all employed mothers.	- Establish and/or increase paid maternity leave; look to countries with successful models for guidance. - Expand family leave benefits to cover all workers and extend benefits to at least six weeks. - Implement tax incentives for employers who provide maternity leave.
Implementation Strategies:	
a) Add maternity leave to the categories of paid leave for federal civil servants.	
b) Develop and implement programs in states to establish a funding mechanism for paid maternity leave.	
14. Ensure that employers establish and maintain comprehensive, high-quality lactation support programs for their employees.	- Establish designated mothers' rooms at worksites. - Allow mothers scheduled breaks of adequate time for milk expression. - Implement tax incentives for employers who provide supportive accommodations. - Enforce regulations that protect breastfeeding support in the workplace.
Implementation Strategies:	
a) Develop resources to help employers comply with federal law that requires employers to provide the time and a place for nursing mothers to express breast milk.	
b) Design and disseminate materials to educate employers about the benefits of providing more comprehensive, high-quality support for breastfeeding employees.	
c) Develop and share innovative solutions to the obstacles to breastfeeding that women face when returning to work in non-office settings.	
d) Promote comprehensive, high-quality lactation support programs as part of a basic employee benefits package.	

15. Expand the use of programs in the workplace that allow lactating mothers to have direct access to their babies. Implementation Strategies: a) Create incentive or recognition programs for businesses that establish, subsidize, and support childcare centers at or near the business site. b) Identify and promote innovative programs that allow mothers to directly breastfeed their babies after they return to work.	- Increase availability of on-site childcare at businesses. - Increase flexibility for new mothers to work from home. - Promote partnerships between employers and nearby childcare facilities. -Implement tax incentives for employers who provide on-site childcare.
16. Ensure that all childcare providers accommodate the needs of breastfeeding mothers and infants. Implementation Strategies: a) Promote adoption of the breastfeeding standards in *Caring for Our Children: National Health and Safety Performance Standards: Guidelines for Out-of-Home Child Care.*	- Educate childcare workers about optimal infant feeding and how to support breastfeeding mothers. - Support childcare workers in learning skills for feeding human milk. - Implement the use of breastfeeding curriculum for childcare centers. - Include actions to support EBF in childcare centers in nationally funded campaigns to fight childhood obesity.

Chapter 6. Monitoring, Evaluation, and Research

The ultimate goal of this review and analysis is to support efforts to increase exclusive breastfeeding. Many innovative interventions and action approaches have been outlined in the previous chapters. These activities will need careful monitoring and evaluation when implemented to ensure successful outcomes. We propose that an iterative systems approach, such as the E-TIERS approach as outlined in Chapter One, be used, ensuring that people, program, outcomes, replicability, and sustainability are all kept in mind at every stage.

Monitoring and evaluation of programs in support of exclusive breastfeeding do not vary substantially from the monitoring and evaluation of any intervention program. The Interstate Collaboration brought together experts in this field from 19 states and large cities, the CDC, Best Fed Beginnings, W. K. Kellogg Foundation, and BFUSA. This group gathered to consider how to support implementation of the Ten Steps to Successful Breastfeeding, a major intervention to increase exclusive breastfeeding. The following draws heavily on the outcomes and final report of the first meeting of the Collaborative (Taylor et al., 2012).

Monitoring is the ongoing collection of data and review of a program's processes and process outcomes to ensure that the plans are being followed. The major goal of monitoring is to assess the occurrence and success of interim steps to ensure that the program design is being followed, but also to allow for mid-course corrections when the outcome of the processes are not as was expected. Monitoring demands clearly defined program benchmarks and the establishment of standardized approaches to the measurement of benchmarks. **Monitoring answers the question: "Are we proceeding as planned?"**

Evaluation, on the other hand, aims to assess if the program achieved its aims and goals. Evaluation outcomes may lead to redesign and adaptation of the entire program approach. **Evaluation answers the question: "Is this program succeeding in achieving the envisioned outcomes and outputs?"**

Research is "studious inquiry or examination; *especially*: investigation or experimentation aimed at the discovery and interpretation of facts, revision of accepted theories or laws in the light of new facts, or practical application of such new or revised theories or laws" (Merriam Webster, 2013). In health research, there generally is an initial hypothesis, and the application of scientific method to consider if the hypothesis can be proven or disproven. **Research answers the question: Is my understanding of**

a possible association between two factors or actions substantiated in scientific study?

Monitoring, evaluation, and research all demand careful definition of the measures, or variables, to be observed. Development of standardized, or minimally, comprehensible definitions of the 1) breastfeeding pattern(s) to be measured, 2) human milk use, and 3) the terms that are related to exclusive breastfeeding success would be a major step towards improvement in the interpretation of interventions.

Monitoring and evaluation also demand carefully crafted objectives that are SMART: **S**pecific, **M**easurable, **A**ttainable, **R**ealistic, and **T**ime dependent. If care is taken to ensure that an objective is SMART, the plan of action is more likely to succeed because it is clear (specific) in what you wish to achieve, you can account for that achievement (measurable), you are realistic in your planning, and you have a timeline, which helps you focus on each step, or task, along the way. Once the objectives are determined for all processes and outcomes, and/or outputs, the manner in which the measures will be collected and reviewed must also be determined. These are all important steps, whether the intervention to be monitored is related to healthcare systems and providers, socioeconomic and sociopolitical factors, or media and marketing. Examples of objectives for monitoring include: 'Training of five groups will be completed by (date) with all groups achieving a grade of at least 85% on post-training test,' or, 'Stakeholders meetings will be held quarterly on the first Monday of each quarter, to review progress against the timeline and to consider if any modification to the timeline is needed." These examples are specific, measurable, hopefully attainable, and realistic (or you will find out in your monitoring and have to carry out a mid-course correction!), and time-defined.

Many examples of SMART objectives may be found in the literature on monitoring and evaluation. Those suggested by the Interstate Collaboration for monitoring of hospital interventions are predicated on the need for:

- Defined benchmarks for internal implementation of innovations.

- Planned discussions and regular review of rates of breastfeeding or rates of other supportive practices. Other suggested benchmarks include not only whether the infant was given formula, but also the age of the infant when the first formula is given, and who gave it.

- All benchmarks should be included in Electronic Medical Records where possible.

- Review at regular meetings of a multi-disciplinary team. The hospital team should include professional leadership at all levels: active involvement of doctors and nurses, hospital and clinical administrators, and, where possible, consumers. In addition, a representative of a nearby hospital with similar interests might be considered.

At the state level, it is recommended that monitoring include:

- Regular reporting on defined benchmarks, such as hospital reports of response to state-level calls for action, collaborative discussions and planning sessions, hospital levels of exclusive breastfeeding, patient satisfaction, shared innovations, and social marketing efforts to support demand creation for patients to have expectations of the Ten Steps.

- Engaging decision-makers and other key stakeholders so that issues of costs and effects, as well as licensing of LCs, may result in greater interest in the program. Inclusion of Medicaid and WIC leadership were common themes and milk banks were mentioned.

Evaluation at the hospital level and state level may occur annually. The annual evaluation addresses whether or not the program achieved the changes that it set out to achieve. Evaluation is strengthened by including stakeholders, such as professional organizations, insurers, media, state epidemiologist and other related state agencies, consumers, and institutions in the review. Evaluation also uses SMART objectives, and generally the evaluation objectives have to do with both achievement of planned outcomes and whether or not those outcomes and outputs resulted in the expected change. For example, you may monitor whether a specific document was prepared in a timely manner, but your evaluation would have to assess if that document was used as expected and whether it achieve the desired change.

The issues suggested by the Interstate Collaboration for evaluation of state level interventions are predicated on the need for:

- Auditing at the state level using existing surveillance instruments, such as immunization surveillance systems.

- Review of ongoing monitoring and the concomitant adjustments, as well as the achievement of planned change.

- Rates of completion of the mPINC survey, with the goal of increasing the number of hospitals and scores.

- Numbers of hospitals striving for state or national designation.

- State or county level exclusive breastfeeding survey data.

Research may exploit data collected for monitoring and evaluation purposes, or may derive from related hypotheses and use independently collected data. In any case, the accuracy of interpretation of research is heavily dependent on the clarity of the definitions of the variables under study. Research findings contribute to evidence-based policy. Mr James Grant, Executive Director of UNICEF, often adapted research findings to underscore his messages. For example:

"Yesterday, merely because mothers were not effectively empowered with the knowledge, were not adequately motivated, and not adequately supported to breastfeed, 3 to 4,000 infants and young children died. Today 3 to 4,000 died; 30 days ago another 3 to 4,000 died."

Source: James P. Grant, Executive Director of UNICEF, in Opening Statement to the WHO/UNICEF Policymakers Meeting on "Breastfeeding in the 1990s: A Global Initiative", Florence, 30 July 1990.

It may be of interest that today, due to increases in EBF globally, this number has been reduced to about 2500-3000.

There is a crying need for more research on every aspect of exclusive breastfeeding. Research is needed at the individual, community, healthcare, state, and national levels on a wide variety of topics. One of the outcomes of the Interstate Collaborative was a series of research questions addressing the Ten Steps. The research questions were edited for clarity, then sent to Collaborative members for comment, and finally to respected experts and researchers for comment and prioritization. This was carried out using a process in which reviewers were asked to consider whether each question was 1) clear, 2) able to be answered through research, 3) likely to support widespread implementation, 4) likely to result in findings that would be readily implementable, and 5) addressing the needs of under-served or under-privileged populations. Reviewers were also asked to rank each question in order of priority. The results were tallied to create a score for each question. The scores were consistently high, and no questions scored so poorly as to indicate exclusion from this set of recommended research questions. The research issues are presented as questions in order of highest to lowest score, as determined by this process. Here, *highest* refers to most clear, most likely to be able to be answered by research, etc. And, *lowest* refers to least clear, least likely to be able to be answered by research, etc. The suggested areas for additional research on this one topic alone were as follows:

Research re: Hospital Practices

1. What is the cost-benefit of Ten Steps implementation at the hospital level?

2. Are there best practices for documenting infant feeding and mother-baby care practices?

3. Does the type of personnel engaged to initiate implementation impact likelihood of progress/success (e.g., administration vs. physician vs. LC; NICU vs. well-baby care, etc.)?

4. Is there a maximally effective ratio of IBCLCs to mother-baby couplets recommended for Ten Steps implementation?

5. Does the use of an outside consultant help speed change?

6. Does a hospital require adding staff to achieve the Ten Steps?

Research re: State Level Programs

1. What is the cost-benefit to Medicaid for reimbursement of lactation support?

2. What are the costs of implementing the Ten Steps vs. the costs of not implementing the Ten Steps at the state/national level?

3. Would state support for increasing the number of IBCLCs improve breastfeeding rates?

4. How many milk banks are needed to address all needs for donor human milk as the supplement of choice for all newborns in the hospital?

Research re: Acceptance of the Ten Steps

1. Can social marketing create consumer demand for the Ten Steps?

2. How does Ten Steps implementation impact patient satisfaction and what factors ensure a positive correlation?

3. What is the best manner to address myths and encourage best practices among health professionals?

4. What is the impact of promoting the Ten Steps on health professionals' attitudes and beliefs about breastfeeding?

5. How do we best address the myths and misperceptions of consumers and patients related to the Ten Steps?

6. What can be done to increase the racial/ethnic diversity of the IBCLCs?

Suggested White Paper Reviews / Policy Analyses

1. How can we reduce formula company influence at all levels?

2. What can state agencies do to motivate hospitals and other state agencies to decide to change?

3. What are the most important things that can be done by State government agencies to support implementation of the Ten Steps? By volunteer coalitions?

4. How does Ten Steps implementation impact hospital staff satisfaction and what factors ensure a positive correlation?

5. What cost-effective approaches exist to assess readiness for change? To identify obstacles to change?

Even this listing, which is for only one topic, is not complete. For example, this listing does not include needed exploration of why, even in Baby-Friendly Hospitals, not all women achieve exclusive breastfeeding success in the hospital, let alone in the days that follow.

Many of programmatic research questions that are raised above merit, minimally, review of the literature and compilation of that review for ready access. Significantly more resources are needed for monitoring, evaluation, and research. We hope that this volume may stimulate possible donors to consider expanding their interest in supporting programs designed to impact exclusive breastfeeding through interventions in health systems, social and political arenas, and in media and marketing.

Our goals for exclusive breastfeeding in the U.S. are outlined in *Healthy People 2020* as 46.2% at three months and 25.5% at six months by 2020, but our goals as supporters of exclusive breastfeeding should aim higher. To achieve these goals, let alone our higher goals, interventions must include the needed monitoring and evaluation, with flexibility to adapt as needed, and the research to help us decide the best paths to success.

Chapter 7. Considerations for Expansion, Replication, and Scaling Up

The previous chapters lay out many areas where action is needed. We do not as yet fully understand all the factors that may influence the context in which each woman lives, loves, works, and worries – her environmental support system. The gaps identified remain to be addressed, but this is not a reason for delay. There are a significant number of well-defined gaps to be addressed and steps to be taken outlined in the previous chapters that will contribute to increases in exclusive breastfeeding. If we address these gaps and take these steps, the result will be increases in exclusive breastfeeding in the U.S., respecting and addressing our special social and societal issues.

If we, then, as a nation, as regions and states, and as groups and individuals, take steps to implement these actions and activities, and achieve increases in exclusive breastfeeding as a result, we will see concomitant decreases in infectious and chronic illnesses, infant and young child mortality, and medical costs for mothers and children from a wide variety of chronic diseases and conditions.

A recent analysis published as a letter in *Pediatrics* (Bonuck, 2007) noted that of the 362 federally funded research projects from 1994-1996 in the area of infant nutrition/ breastfeeding/lactation, 31 (or 8.6%) had as a goal to increase breastfeeding. The author carried out a similar analysis of the 422 projects funded in a more recent period, 2003-2006, and found that only four, or less than 1%, specified a direct or indirect goal of increasing breastfeeding.

It may also be of concern that the research literature on breastfeeding may be shifting away from examining exclusive breastfeeding, *per se*. According to PubMed search engines, the percent of papers on breastfeeding that included "exclusive breastfeeding" was about 84% in the last decade. While this remains a significant proportion of all, the proportion the previous two decades, ending in 2002, was 94.4%, and in the decades prior to 1982, the percent was greater than 98%.

During this same decade, the quantity and quality of findings on the importance of breastfeeding, especially exclusive breastfeeding, for health and survival have increased significantly. Anything less than exclusive breastfeeding clearly carries risks.

Single pilot programs are simply not sufficient to achieve the needed changes in support for women to succeed in exclusive breastfeeding for six months. If we return to the constructs presented in Chapter One (Planning for Action: Influence and Timing, and the 'E-TIERs' Approach), especially the E-TIERS approach, we can see that replication and sustainability are equally, if not more important, than carrying out a successful pilot effort. Evaluation, preparation for replication, and designing for sustainable scale-up must be part of the consideration, even in design of that first pilot effort.

Chapter 8. Next Steps

Progress on exclusive breastfeeding has been remarkable, both in the U.S. and worldwide; however, a significant increase in attention to this issue is essential for any further success. If we are to succeed in supporting women to decide to exclusively breastfeed, and to succeed with this decision, we must address the following:

- Need for better definitions for exclusive breastfeeding, and breastfeeding in general. As long as vastly different, or no definitions of the pattern of breastfeeding under discussion is included in program design, monitoring, evaluation, or research, it will be very difficult to determine exactly what changes are needed to achieve exclusive breastfeeding.

- Need for ongoing literature review, as well as clinical and program research, in the areas of health, society and policy, and media and marketing. There remains a pressing need for ongoing systematic review of the literature with attention to the definitions and other variables in use. Until there is some comparability in the definitions, conclusions drawn may be apparently contradictory, when the findings may, in fact, be compatible.

- Need for implementation of the 20 action areas laid out in the Surgeon General's report. These action areas are reflective of the international strategies outlined in *Innocenti*, *Global Strategy*, and *Innocenti +15*. However, those strategies are predicated on countries' acceptance of the Convention of the Rights of the Child, The Convention to End Discrimination Against Women, and the guidance of the International Labor Organization, which calls for a minimum of 14 weeks paid maternity leave, as well as workplace accommodation upon return to work.

- Need for increased understanding of the physiology and maintenance of milk supply. We remain unclear why some women are not able to achieve full, exclusive breastfeeding. Logically, the vast majority of women are able to fully breastfeed, or our species would not have survived over the millennia. This may be due to physiological, psychological, or practical barriers. We are not fully on top of these issues and concerns; more work is essential for forward momentum.

- Need for significant and sustainable changes in local, city, state, and national policies. Now that the Surgeon General has issued a *Call to Action* that reflects international goals, it is time for our state and national policies to do the same as other nations, including addressing the need for paid maternity leave and workplace accommodation, support for grassroots innovations, health systems change, and political confirmation that breastfeeding is an essential component of our desire to raise more healthy generations to come.

Given these findings, this book calls for a broadening of the awareness of the real changes needed to increase exclusive breastfeeding. Increased federal, state, and other funding for health providers, researchers, and planners for social, economic, and workplace accommodation and paid leave, for related political action, and towards media and marketing regulation is necessary if we are truly dedicated to enabling women to decide on the feeding course that supports health and survival, and to succeed in establishing six months of exclusive breastfeeding as the normative feeding pattern in the United States.

References

Al-Sahab, B., Lanes, A., Feldman, M., & Tamim, H. (2010). Prevalence and predictors of 6-month exclusive breastfeeding among Canadian women: a national survey. *BMC pediatrics, 10*(1), 20.

Alikasifoglu, M., Erginoz, E., Gur, E. T., Baltas, Z., Beker, B., & Arvas, A. (2001). Factors influencing the duration of exclusive breastfeeding in a group of Turkish women. *Journal of Human Lactation, 17*(3), 220.

American Academy of Family Physicians. (2008). *Family physicians supporting breastfeeding* (position paper). Retrieved from: http://www.aafp.org/online/en/home/policy/policies/b/breastfeedingpositionpaper.htm

American College of Obstetricians and Gynecologists, Committee on Health Care for Underserved Women. (2007). ACOG Committee Opinion No. 361: Breastfeeding: maternal and infant aspects. *Obstet Gynecol, 109*(2 Pt 1), 479-480.

American College of Preventive Medicine. (2012). *Resolution on Breastfeeding*. Retrieved from: http://www.acpm.org/?Policy_Issues

Anderson, A. K., Damio, G., Young, S., Chapman, D. J., & Perez-Escamilla, R. (2005). A randomized trial assessing the efficacy of peer counseling on exclusive breastfeeding in a predominantly Latina low-income community. *Archives of Pediatrics and Adolescent Medicine, 159*(9), 836.

Association of Women's Health Obstetric and Neonatal Nurses. (2007). *Breastfeeding support: Prenatal care through the first year. Evidence-based clinical practical guideline.* (Second Ed.). Washington, D.C.: Association of Women's Health, Obstetric and Neonatal Nurses.

Baby Friendly USA. (2012). *Baby-friendly hospitals and birth centers.* Retrieved from http://www.babyfriendlyusa.org/eng/03.html

Bai, Y., Middlestadt, S. E., Peng, C. Y. J., & Fly, A. D. (2010). Predictors of continuation of exclusive breastfeeding for the first six months of life. *Journal of Human Lactation, 26*(1), 26-34.

Bai, Y., Wunderlich, S. M., & Fly, A. D. (2011). Predicting intentions to continue exclusive breastfeeding for 6 months: A comparison among racial/ethnic groups. *Matern Child Health J, 15*(8):1257-64.

Baker, M., & Milligan, K. (2008). Maternal employment, breastfeeding, and health: Evidence from maternity leave mandates. *Journal of Health Economics, 27*(4), 871-887.

Balkam, J. A., Cadwell, K., & Fein, S. B. (2011). Effect of components of a workplace lactation program on breastfeeding duration among employees of a public-sector employer. *Matern Child Health J, 15*(5), 677-683. doi: 10.1007/s10995-010-0620-9

Ball, T. M., & Bennett, D. M. (2001). The economic impact of breastfeeding. *Pediatric Clinics of North America, 48*(1), 253-262.

Bartick, M., & Reinhold, A. (2010). The burden of suboptimal breastfeeding in the United States: A pediatric cost analysis. *Pediatrics, 125*(5), e1048-e1056.

Baumslag, N., & Michels, D. L. (1995). Milk, money and madness: Culture and politics of breastfeeding. *Recherche, 67,* 02.

Benjamin, S. E., Taveras, E. M., Cradock, A. L., Walker, E. M., Slining, M. M., & Gillman, M. W. (2009). State and regional variation in regulations related to feeding infants in child care. *Pediatrics, 124*(1), e104-e111.

Bernaix, L. W., Beaman, M. L., Schmidt, C. A., Harris, J. K., & Miller, L. M. (2010). Success of an educational intervention on maternal/newborn nurses' breastfeeding knowledge and attitudes. *Journal of Obstetric, Gynecologic, & Neonatal Nursing, 39*(6), 658-666.

Binstock, M. A., & Wolde-Tsadik, G. (1995). Alternative prenatal care. Impact of reduced visit frequency, focused visits and continuity of care. *J Reprod Med, 40*(7), 507-512.

Biro, M. A., Sutherland, G. A., Yelland, J. S., Hardy, P., & Brown, S. J. (2011). In-hospital formula supplementation of breastfed babies: A population-based survey. *Birth, 38*(4): 302-310.

Blyth, R., Creedy, D. K., Dennis, C. L., Moyle, W., Pratt, J., & De Vries, S. M. (2002). Effect of maternal confidence on breastfeeding duration: An application of breastfeeding self-efficacy theory. *Birth, 29*(4), 278-284.

Bonuck, K. (2007). Paucity of evidence-based research on how to achieve the Healthy People 2012 goal of exclusive breastfeeding. *Pediatrics, 120*(1), 248-249.

Broadfoot, M., Britten, J., Tappin, D., & MacKenzie, J. (2005). The baby friendly hospital initiative and breast feeding rates in Scotland. *Archives of Disease in Childhood. Fetal and Neonatal Edition, 90*(2), F114.

Brown, A., & Lee, M. (2011). An exploration of the attitudes and experiences of mothers in the United Kingdom who chose to breastfeed exclusively for 6 months postpartum. *Breastfeeding Medicine, 6*(4), 197-204.

Cattaneo, A. (2004). *Protection, promotion and support of breastfeeding in Europe: A blueprint for action.* Trieste, Italy: Unit for Health Services Research and International Health.

Centers for Disease Control and Prevention. (2005). *Infant Feeding Practices Study II data results.* Retrieved from: http://www.cdc.gov/ifps/results/index.htm

Centers for Disease Control and Prevention. (2011a). *Breastfeeding report card - United States, 2011.* Retrieved from: http://www.cdc.gov/breastfeeding/data/reportcard/reportcard2011.htm

Centers for Disease Control and Prevention. (2010). *Racial and ethnic differences in breastfeeding initiation and duration, by state---National Immunization Survey, United States, 2004--2008.* Retrieved from: http://www.cdc.gov/mmwr/preview/mmwrhtml/mm5911a2.htm

Centers for Disease Control and Prevention. (2011b). Update to CDC's U.S. Medical Eligibility Criteria for Contraceptive Use, 2010: Revised recommendations for the use of contraceptive methods during the postpartum period. *MMWR Morb Mortal Wkly Rep, 60*(26), 878-883.

Cernadas, J. M. C., Noceda, G., Barrera, L., Martinez, A. M., & Garsd, A. (2003). Maternal and perinatal factors influencing the duration of exclusive breastfeeding during the first 6 months of life. *Journal of Human Lactation, 19*(2), 136.

Chalmers, B., Levitt, C., Heaman, M., O'Brien, B., Sauve, R., & Kaczorowski, J. (2009). Breastfeeding rates and hospital breastfeeding practices in Canada: A national survey of women. *Birth, 36*(2), 122-132.

Chapman, D. J., Damio, G., Young, S., & Perez-Escamilla, R. (2004). Effectiveness of breastfeeding peer counseling in a low-income, predominantly Latina population: A randomized controlled trial. *Archives of Pediatrics and Adolescent Medicine, 158*(9), 897.

Chapman, D. J., & Perez-Escamilla, R. (1999). Identification of risk factors for delayed onset of lactation. *Journal of the American Dietetic Association, 99*(4), 450-454.

Chen, B. A., Reeves, M. F., Creinin, M. D., & Schwarz, E. B. (2011). Postplacental or delayed levonorgestrel intrauterine device insertion and breast-feeding duration. *Contraception, 84*(5):499-504.

Chien, L. Y., Tai, C. J., Chu, K. H., Ko, Y. L., & Chiu, Y. C. (2007). The number of Baby Friendly hospital practices experienced by mothers is positively associated with breastfeeding: A questionnaire survey. *Int J Nurs Stud, 44*(7), 1138-1146. doi: 10.1016/j.ijnurstu.2006.05.015

Chung, M., Raman, G., Trikalinos, T., Lau, J., & Ip, S. (2008). Interventions in primary care to promote breastfeeding: An evidence review for the US Preventive Services Task Force. *Annals of Internal Medicine, 149*(8), 565-582.

Clifford, T. J., Campbell, M. K., Speechley, K. N., & Gorodzinsky, F. (2006). Factors influencing full breastfeeding in a southwestern Ontario community: Assessments at 1 week and at 6 months postpartum. *Journal of Human Lactation, 22*(3), 292.

Cohen, R. J., Brown, K. H., Rivera, L. L., & Dewey, K. G. (1999). Promoting exclusive breastfeeding for 4-6 months in Honduras: Attitudes of mothers and barriers to compliance. *Journal of Human Lactation, 15*(1), 9.

Cross-Barnet, C., Augustyn, M., Gross, S., Resnik, A., & Paige, D. (2012). Long-term breastfeeding support: Failing mothers in need. *Maternal and Child Health Journal, 16*(9):1926-32.

Dabritz, H. A., Hinton, B. G., & Babb, J. (2010). Maternal hospital experiences associated with breastfeeding at 6 months in a northern California county. *Journal of Human Lactation, 26*(3), 274-285.

Dall'Oglio, I., Salvatori, G., Bonci, E., Nantini, B., D'Agostino, G., & Dotta, A. (2007). Breastfeeding promotion in neonatal intensive care unit: Impact of a new program toward a BFHI for high-risk infants. *Acta Paediatr, 96*(11), 1626-1631. doi: 10.1111/j.1651-2227.2007.00495.x

Darmstadt, G. L., Bhutta, Z. A., Cousens, S., Adam, T., Walker, N., & de Bernis, L. (2005). Evidence-based, cost-effective interventions: How many newborn babies can we save? *Lancet, 365*(9463), 977-988. doi: 10.1016/s0140-6736(05)71088-6

Davis, L. G., Riedmann, G. L., Sapiro, M., Minogue, J. P., Kazer, R. R. (1994). Cesarean section rates in low-risk private patients managed by certified nurse-midwives and obstetricians. *J Nurse Midwifery, 39*(2):91-7.

Dearden, K. A., Quan, L., Do, M., Marsh, D., Pachón, H., Schroeder, D., & Lang, T. (2002). Work outside the home is the primary barrier to exclusive breastfeeding in rural Viet Nam: Insights from mothers who exclusively breastfed and worked. *Food Nutr Bull, 23*(4 Suppl), 99-106.

Declercq, E., Labbok, M. H., Sakala, C., & O'Hara, M. A. (2009). Hospital practices and women's likelihood of fulfilling their intention to exclusively breastfeed. *American Journal of Public Health, 99*(5), 929.

Declercq, E. M., Sakala, C., Corry, M. P., & Applebaum, S. (2007). Listening to Mothers II: Report of the Second National U.S. Survey of Women's Childbearing Experiences: Conducted January-February 2006 for Childbirth Connection by Harris Interactive(R) in partnership with Lamaze International. *J Perinat Educ, 16*(4), 15-17. doi: 10.1624/105812407x244778

Dennis, C. L., & Faux, S. (1999). Development and psychometric testing of the Breastfeeding Self-Efficacy Scale. *Res Nurs Health, 22*(5), 399-409.

Dennis, C. L., & McQueen, K. (2009). The relationship between infant-feeding outcomes and postpartum depression: A qualitative systematic review. *Pediatrics, 123*(4), e736-e751.

Dewey, K. G., Nommsen-Rivers, L. A., Heinig, M. J., & Cohen, R. J. (2003). Risk factors for suboptimal infant breastfeeding behavior, delayed onset of lactation, and excess neonatal weight loss. *Pediatrics, 112*(3), 607.

DHHS Centers for Disease Control and Prevention. (2012). Breastfeeding: Data and statistics: National Immunization Survey (NIS). Retrieved from: http://www.cdc.gov/breastfeeding/data/NIS_data/index.htm

DHHS Healthy People 2010. (2000). *Maternal, infant, and child health*. (Archived) Retrieved from: http://www.healthypeople.gov/2010/

DHHS Office on Women's Health. (August 2012). *National Breastfeeding Awareness Campaign*. Retrieved from: http://womenshealth.gov/breastfeeding/government-in-action/national-breastfeeding-campaign/

DiGirolamo, A. M., Grummer-Strawn, L. M., & Fein, S. B. (2008). Effect of maternity-care practices on breastfeeding. *Pediatrics, 122*(Supplement 2), S43-S49.

Dillaway, H. E., & Douma, M. E. (2004). Are pediatric offices "supportive" of breastfeeding? Discrepancies between mothers' and healthcare professionals' reports. *Clin Pediatr (Phila), 43*(5), 417-430.

Donnelly, A., Snowden, H., Renfrew, M., & Woolridge, M. (2001). Commercial hospital discharge packs for breastfeeding women. *Birth, 28*(1), 63-64.

Dungy, C. I., Christensen-Szalanski, J., Losch, M., & Russell, D. (1992). Effect of discharge samples on duration of breast-feeding. *Pediatrics, 90*(2), 233.

Dusdieker, L. B., Dungy, C. I., & Losch, M. E. (2006). Prenatal office practices regarding infant feeding choices. *Clinical Pediatrics, 45*(9), 841-845.

Edmond, K. M., Zandoh, C., Quigley, M. A., Amenga-Etego, S., Owusu-Agyei, S., & Kirkwood, B. R. (2006). Delayed breastfeeding initiation increases risk of neonatal mortality. *Pediatrics, 117*(3), e380-386. doi: 10.1542/peds.2005-1496

Eidelman, A. I., Schanler, R. J., Johnston, M., Landers, S., Noble, L., Szucs, K., & Viehmann, L. (2012). Breastfeeding and the use of human milk. *Pediatrics, 129*(3), e827-e841.

Emmett, P. M., & Rogers, I. S. (1997). Properties of human milk and their relationship with maternal nutrition. *Early Hum Dev, 49* Suppl, S7-28.

Fein, S. B., Mandal, B., & Roe, B. E. (2008). Success of strategies for combining employment and breastfeeding. *Pediatrics, 122*(Supplement 2), S56-S62.

Fein, S. B., & Roe, B. (1998). The effect of work status on initiation and duration of breast-feeding. *American Journal of Public Health, 88*(7), 1042.

Feldman-Winter, L. B., Schanler, R. J., O'Connor, K. G., & Lawrence, R. A. (2008). Pediatricians and the promotion and support of breastfeeding. *Archives of Pediatrics and Adolescent Medicine, 162*(12), 1142.

Feldman-Winter L. (2012) The AAP updates its policy on breastfeeding and reaches consensus on recommended duration of exclusive breastfeeding. *Journal of Human Lactation, 28*(2):116-7.

Flores, M., Pasquel, M. R., Maulén, I., & Rivera, J. (2005). Exclusive breastfeeding in 3 rural localities in Mexico. *Journal of Human Lactation, 21*(3), 276-283.

Frank, D. A., Wirtz, S. J., Sorenson, J. R., & Heeren, T. (1987). Commercial discharge packs and breast-feeding counseling: Effects on infant-feeding practices in a randomized trial. *Pediatrics, 80*(6), 845.

Gartner, L., Black, L., Eaton, A., Lawrence, R., Naylor, A., Neifert, M., . . . Piovanetti, Y. (1997). Breastfeeding and the use of human milk. *Pediatrics, 100*(6), 1035-1039.

Gartner, L. M., Morton, J., Lawrence, R. A., Naylor, A. J., O'Hare, D., Schanler, R. J., & Eidelman, A. I. (2005). Breastfeeding and the use of human milk. *Pediatrics, 115*(2), 496.

Gatti, L. (2008). Maternal perceptions of insufficient milk supply in breastfeeding. *Journal of Nursing Scholarship, 40*(4), 355-363.

Geraghty, S. R., Riddle, S. W., & Shaikh, U. (2008). The breastfeeding mother and the pediatrician. *Journal of Human Lactation, 24*(3), 335-339.

Gilmour, C., Hall, H., McIntyre, M., Gillies, L., & Harrison, B. (2009). Factors associated with early breastfeeding cessation in Frankston, Victoria: A descriptive study. *Breastfeeding Review: Professional Publication of the Nursing Mothers' Association of Australia, 17*(2), 13.

Gray, R. H., Campbell, O. M., Apelo, R., Eslami, S. S., Zacur, H., Ramos, R. M., . . . Labbok, M. H. (1990). Risk of ovulation during lactation. *Lancet, 335*(8680), 25-29.

Greiner, T., & Latham, M. C. (1982). The influence of infant food advertising on infant feeding practices in St. Vincent. *International Journal of Health Services, 12*(1), 53-75.

Grummer-Strawn, L. (2006). Maternal & Child Health Branch, Division of Nutrition and Physical Activity, United States CDC and Prevention. Letter to the Massachusetts Public Health Council. 2006 Apr 26.

Gurtcheff, S. E., Turok, D. K., Stoddard, G., Murphy, P. A., Gibson, M., & Jones, K. P. (2011). Lactogenesis after early postpartum use of the contraceptive implant: A randomized controlled trial. *Obstetrics & Gynecology, 117*(5), 1114.

Halderman, L. D., & Nelson, A. L. (2002). Impact of early postpartum administration of progestin-only hormonal contraceptives compared with nonhormonal contraceptives on short-term breast-feeding patterns. *Am J Obstet Gynecol, 186*(6), 1250-1256; discussion 1256-1258.

Hawkins, S. S., Griffiths, L. J., Dezateux, C., & Law, C. (2007). Maternal employment and breastfeeding initiation: Findings from the Millennium Cohort Study. *Paediatric and Perinatal Epidemiology, 21*(3), 242-247.

Hilson, J. A., Rasmussen, K. M., & Kjolhede, C. L. (2006). Excessive weight gain during pregnancy is associated with earlier termination of breast-feeding among white women. *The Journal of Nutrition, 136*(1), 140.

Hopkinson, J., & Konefal Gallagher, M. (2009). Assignment to a hospital-based breastfeeding clinic and exclusive breastfeeding among immigrant Hispanic mothers: A randomized, controlled trial. *Journal of Human Lactation, 25*(3), 287.

Hörnell, A., Hofvander, Y., & Kylberg, E. (2001). Solids and formula: Association with pattern and duration of breastfeeding. *Pediatrics, 107*(3), e38.

Howard, C. R., Howard, F. M., Lanphear, B., Eberly, S., deBlieck, E. A., Oakes, D., & Lawrence, R. A. (2003). Randomized clinical trial of pacifier use and bottle-feeding or cupfeeding and their effect on breastfeeding. *Pediatrics, 111*(3), 511.

Howard, C. R., Weitzman, M., Lawrence, R., & Howard, F. M. (1994). Antenatal formula advertising: Another potential threat to breast-feeding. *Pediatrics, 94*(1), 102.

Institute for Clinical Systems Improvement. (2012). *Health care guideline: Routine prenatal care*. Retrieved from: https://www.icsi.org/guidelines__more/catalog_guidelines_and_more/catalog_guidelines/catalog_womens_health_guidelines/prenatal/

International Board of Lactation Consultant Examiners. (2011). *Steps to becoming an IBCLC*. Retrieved from: http://americas.iblce.org/steps-to-becoming-an-ibclc

Ip, S., Chung, M., Raman, G., Chew, P., Magula, N., DeVine, D., . . . Lau, J. (2007). Breastfeeding and maternal and infant health outcomes in developed countries. *Evid Rep Technol Assess (Full Rep)*(153), 1-186.

James, D. C., & Lessen, R. (2009). Position of the American Dietetic Association: Promoting and supporting breastfeeding. *J Am Diet Assoc, 109*(11), 1926-1942.

Jelliffe, D.B. (1972). Commerciogenic malnutrition? *Nutrition Review, 30*(9):199-205.

Johnson, K., Posner, S. F., Biermann, J., Cordero, J. F., Atrash, H. K., Parker, C. S., . . . Curtis, M. G. (2006). Recommendations to improve preconception health and health care--United States. A report of the CDC/ATSDR Preconception Care Work Group and the Select Panel on Preconception Care. *MMWR Recomm Rep, 55*(RR-6), 1-23.

Jones, G., Steketee, R. W., Black, R. E., Bhutta, Z. A., & Morris, S. S. (2003). How many child deaths can we prevent this year? *Lancet, 362*(9377), 65-71. doi: 10.1016/s0140-6736(03)13811-1

Kelly, Y., & Watt, R. (2005). Breast-feeding initiation and exclusive duration at 6 months by social class—results from the Millennium Cohort Study. *Public Health Nutrition, 8*(04), 417-421.

Kennedy K, Bellagio Consensus Statement. (1988). Breastfeeding as a family planning method. *Lancet,* ii:1204-1205.

Killien, M. G. (2005). The role of social support in facilitating postpartum women's return to employment. *J Obstet Gynecol Neonatal Nurs, 34*(5), 639-646. doi: 10.1177/0884217505280192

Kronborg, H., & Væth, M. (2004). The influence of psychosocial factors on the duration of breastfeeding. *Scandinavian Journal of Public Health, 32*(3), 210-216.

Kronborg, H., & Væth, M. (2009). How are effective breastfeeding technique and pacifier use related to breastfeeding problems and breastfeeding duration? *Birth, 36*(1), 34-42.

Kronborg, H., Væth, M., Olsen, J., Iversen, L., & Harder, I. (2007). Effect of early postnatal breastfeeding support: A cluster-randomized community based trial. *Acta Paediatrica, 96*(7), 1064-1070.

Kruske, S., Schmied, V., & Cook, M. (2007). The 'Early bird' gets the breastmilk: Findings from an evaluation of combined professional and peer support groups to improve breastfeeding duration in the first eight weeks after birth. *Maternal & Child Nutrition, 3*(2), 108-119.

Kurinij, N., & Shiono, P. H. (1991). Early formula supplementation of breast-feeding. *Pediatrics, 88*(4), 745.

Labbok, M. H. (1994). Breastfeeding as a women's issue: Conclusions and consensus, complementary concerns, and next actions. *Int J Gynaecol Obstet, 47 Suppl,* S55-61.

Labbok, M. H. (2012) Global Baby-Friendly Hospital Initiative monitoring data: Update and discussion. *Breastfeeding Medicine,7*(4):210-222.

Labbok, M. H., Clark, D., & Goldman, A. S. (2004). Breastfeeding: Maintaining an irreplaceable immunological resource. *Nat Rev Immunol, 4*(7), 565-572. doi: 10.1038/nri1393

Labbok, M. H., Hight-Laukaran, V., Peterson, A. E., Fletcher, V., von Hertzen, H., & Van Look, P. F. (1997). Multicenter study of the Lactational Amenorrhea Method (LAM): I. Efficacy, duration, and implications for clinical application. *Contraception, 55*(6), 327-336.

Labbok, M. H., & Krasovec, K. (1990). Toward consistency in breastfeeding definitions. *Studies in family planning, 21*(4), 226-230.

Li, R., Darling, N., Maurice, E., Barker, L., & Grummer-Strawn, L. M. (2005). Breastfeeding rates in the United States by characteristics of the child, mother, or family: The 2002 National Immunization Survey. *Pediatrics, 115*(1), e31-e37.

Li, R., Fein, S. B., Chen, J., & Grummer-Strawn, L. M. (2008). Why mothers stop breastfeeding: Mothers' self-reported reasons for stopping during the first year. *Pediatrics, 122*(Supplement 2), S69-S76.

Li, R., Fridinger, F., & Grummer-Strawn, L. (2002). Public perceptions on breastfeeding constraints. *Journal of Human Lactation, 18*(3), 227-235.

Li, R., Rock, V. J., & Grummer-Strawn, L. (2007). Changes in public attitudes toward breastfeeding in the United States, 1999-2003. *Journal of the American Dietetic Association, 107*(1), 122-127.

Liebert, M. (2008). Academy of Breastfeeding Medicine. Position on breastfeeding. *Breastfeeding Medicine, 3*(4), 267-270.

Lu, M. C., Kotelchuck, M., Culhane, J. F., Hobel, C. J., Klerman, L. V., & Thorp, J. M., Jr. (2006). Preconception care between pregnancies: The content of internatal care. *Matern Child Health J, 10*(5 Suppl), S107-122. doi: 10.1007/s10995-006-0118-7

Ludvigsson, J. F., & Ludvigsson, J. (2005). Socioeconomic determinants, maternal smoking and coffee consumption, and exclusive breastfeeding in 10 205 children. *Acta Paediatrica, 94*(9), 1310-1319.

Maia, C., Brandao, R., Roncalli, A., & Maranhao, H. (2011). Length of stay in a neonatal intensive care unit and its association with low rates of exclusive breastfeeding in very low birth weight infants. *J Matern Fetal Neonatal Med, 24*(6), 774-777. doi: 10.3109/14767058.2010.520046

Mannel, R., & Mannel, R. S. (2006). Staffing for hospital lactation programs: Recommendations from a tertiary care teaching hospital. *J Hum Lact, 22*(4), 409-417. doi: 10.1177/0890334406294166

Martens, P. J. (2000). Does breastfeeding education affect nursing staff beliefs, exclusive breastfeeding rates, and Baby-Friendly Hospital Initiative compliance? The experience of a small, rural Canadian hospital. *Journal of Human lactation, 16*(4), 309.

Martin, J. A., Hamilton, B. E., Sutton, P. D., Ventura, S. J., Mathews, T. J., & Osterman, M. J. (2010). Births: Final data for 2008. *Natl Vital Stat Rep, 59*(1), 1, 3-71.

Martin, J. A., Hamilton, B. E., Sutton, P. D., Ventura, S. J., Menacker, F., & Kirmeyer, S. (2006). Births: Final data for 2004. *Natl Vital Stat Rep, 55*(1), 1-101.

Martin, J. A., Hamilton, B. E., Ventura, S. J., Osterman, M. J., Kirmeyer, S., Mathews, T. J., & Wilson, E. C. (2011). Births: Final Data for 2009. National Vital Statistics Reports, 60(1).

Merriam Webster (m-w.com). Research. *Encyclopædia Britannica.* Retrieved from: http://www.merriam-webster.com/dictionary/research

Merten, S., Dratva, J., & Ackermann-Liebrich, U. (2005). Do baby-friendly hospitals influence breastfeeding duration on a national level? *Pediatrics, 116*(5), e702.

Mistry, Y., Freedman, M., Sweeney, K., & Hollenbeck, C. (2008). Infant-feeding practices of low-income Vietnamese American women. *Journal of Human Lactation, 24*(4), 406-414.

Montgomery, D. L., & Splett, P. L. (1997). Economic benefit of breast-feeding infants enrolled in WIC. *J Am Diet Assoc, 97*(4), 379-385. doi: 10.1016/s0002-8223(97)00094-1

Moos, M. K. (2004). Preconceptional health promotion: Progress in changing a prevention paradigm. *J Perinat Neonatal Nurs, 18*(1), 2-13.

Moos, M. K. (2006). Prenatal care: Limitations and opportunities. *J Obstet Gynecol Neonatal Nurs, 35*(2), 278-285. doi: 10.1111/j.1552-6909.2006.00039.x

Morrow, A. L., Guerrero, M. L., Shults, J., Calva, J. J., Lutter, C., Bravo, J., . . . Butterfoss, F. D. (1999). Efficacy of home-based peer counselling to promote exclusive breastfeeding: A randomised controlled trial. *The Lancet, 353*(9160), 1226-1231.

Morton, J., Hall, J. Y., Wong, R. J., Thairu, L., Benitz, W. E., & Rhine, W. D. (2009). Combining hand techniques with electric pumping increases milk production in mothers of preterm infants. *J Perinatol, 29*(11), 757-764. doi: 10.1038/jp.2009.87

Morton, J., Wong, R. J., Hall, J. Y., Pang, W. W., Lai, C. T., Lui, J., . . . Rhine, W. D. (2012). Combining hand techniques with electric pumping increases the caloric content of milk in mothers of preterm infants. *J Perinatol, 32*(10), 791-796. doi: 10.1038/jp.2011.195

National Association of Pediatric Nurse Practitioners. (2001). Position statement on breastfeeding. *J Pediatr Health Care, 15*(5), 22A.

Osband, Y. B., Altman, R. L., Patrick, P. A., & Edwards, K. S. (2011). Breastfeeding education and support services offered to pediatric residents in the US. *Academic Pediatrics, 11*(1), 75-79.

Osis, M. J. D., Duarte, G. A., Pádua, K. S., Hardy, E., Sandoval, L. E. M., & Bento, S. F. (2004). Exclusive breastfeeding among working women with free daycare available at workplace. *Revista de Saúde Pública, 38*(2), 172-179.

Parkinson, J., Russell-Bennett, R., & Previte, J. (2010). *The role of mother-centered factors influencing the complex social behaviour of breastfeeding: Social support and self-efficacy.* Paper presented at the Australian and New Zealand Marketing Conference: Doing more with Less, Christchurch, New Zealand.

Parry, K., Taylor, E., Hall-Dardess, P., Walker, M., & Labbok, M. (2013). Understanding women's interpretation of infant formula advertising. *Under Review: Birth: Issues in Perinatal Care.*

Pechlivani, F., Vassilakou, T., Sarafidou, J., Zachou, T., Anastasiou, C. A., & Sidossis, L. S. (2005). Prevalence and determinants of exclusive breastfeeding during hospital stay in the area of Athens, Greece. *Acta Paediatrica, 94*(7), 928-934.

Perez, A., Vela, P., Potter, R., & Masnick, G. (1971). Timing and sequence of resuming ovulation and menstruation after childbirth. *Pop Stud*, 25(3):491-503.

Petrova, A., Hegyi, T., & Mehta, R. (2007). Maternal race/ethnicity and one-month exclusive breastfeeding in association with the in-hospital feeding modality. *Breastfeeding Medicine, 2*(2), 92-98.

Pharmaceutical Research and Manufacturers of America. (2012). *PHhRMA Code on Interactions with Healthcare Professionals.* Retrieved from: http://www.phrma.org/about/principles-guidelines/code-interactions-healthcare-professionals

Philipp, B. L., Malone, K. L., Cimo, S., & Merewood, A. (2003). Sustained breastfeeding rates at a US baby-friendly hospital. *Pediatrics, 112*(3), e234-e236.

Radford, A. (1992). The ecological impact of bottle feeding. *Breastfeeding Review, 2*(1), 204-208.

Raisler, J., Alexander, C., & O'Campo, P. (1999). Breast-feeding and infant illness: A dose-response relationship? *Am J Public Health, 89*(1), 25-30.

Raju, T. (2006). Continued barriers for breast-feeding in public and the workplace. *The Journal of Pediatrics, 148*(5), 677.

Renfrew, M. J., Craig, D., Dyson, L., McCormick, F., Rice, S., King, S. E., . . . Williams, A. F. (2009). Breastfeeding promotion for infants in neonatal units: A systematic review and economic analysis. *Health Technol Assess, 13*(40), 1-146, iii-iv. doi: 10.3310/hta13400

Rosenberg, K. D., Eastham, C. A., Kasehagen, L. J., & Sandoval, A. P. (2008). Marketing infant formula through hospitals: The impact of commercial hospital discharge packs on breastfeeding. *American Journal of Public Health, 98*(2), 290.

Rowe⊠Murray, H. J., & Fisher, J. R. W. (2002). Baby friendly hospital practices: Cesarean section is a persistent barrier to early initiation of breastfeeding. *Birth, 29*(2), 124-131.

Ruchala, P. L., & Halstead, L. (1994). The postpartum experience of low-risk women: A time of adjustment and change. *Maternal-Child Nursing Journal, 22*(3), 83-89.

Russo, C. A., Wier, L., & Steiner, C. (2006). Hospitalizations related to childbirth, 2006: Statistical brief #71, *Healthcare cost and utilization project (HCUP) statistical briefs.* Rockville MD.

Scott, J. A., Binns, C. W., Oddy, W. H., & Graham, K. I. (2006). Predictors of breastfeeding duration: Evidence from a cohort study. *Pediatrics, 117*(4), e646.

Scott, J. A., Landers, M. C. G., Hughes, R. M., & Binns, C. W. (2001). Psychosocial factors associated with the abandonment of breastfeeding prior to hospital discharge. *Journal of Human Lactation, 17*(1), 24.

Semenic, S., Loiselle, C., & Gottlieb, L. (2008). Predictors of the duration of exclusive breastfeeding among first-time mothers. *Research in Nursing & Health, 31*(5), 428-441.

Sherriff, N., & Hall, V. (2011). Engaging and supporting fathers to promote breastfeeding: A new role for Health Visitors? *Scandinavian Journal of Caring Sciences, 25*(3), 467-475.

Sikorski, J., Renfrew, M. J., Pindoria, S., & Wade, A. (2003). Support for breastfeeding mothers: A systematic review. *Paediatric and perinatal epidemiology, 17*(4), 407-417.

Simopoulos, A., & Grave, G. (1984). Factors associated with the choice and duration of infant-feeding practice. *Pediatrics 74*(4, pt. 2), 603-614.

Spiby, H., McCormick, F., Wallace, L., Renfrew, M. J., D'Souza, L., & Dyson, L. (2009). A systematic review of education and evidence-based practice interventions with health professionals and breast feeding counsellors on duration of breast feeding. *Midwifery, 25*(1), 50-61.

Su, L. L., Chong, Y. S., Chan, Y. H., Chan, Y. S., Fok, D., Tun, K. T., . . . Rauff, M. (2007). Antenatal education and postnatal support strategies for improving rates of exclusive breast feeding: Randomised controlled trial. *BMJ, 335*(7620), 596.

Taveras, E. M., Li, R., Grummer-Strawn, L., Richardson, M., Marshall, R., Rêgo, V. H., . . . Lieu, T. A. (2004). Opinions and practices of clinicians associated with continuation of exclusive breastfeeding. *Pediatrics, 113*(4), e283.

Taylor, E., Colgan, B., Labbok, M., with members of the Interstate Collaborative. (2012). *Findings and Recommendations from the 2011 Meeting of the The Interstate Collaborative to Support Widespread Implementation of the Ten Steps to Successful Breastfeeding.* Chapel Hill, NC: Carolina Global Breastfeeding Institute.

Taylor, J. S., & Cabral, H. J. (2002). Are women with an unintended pregnancy less likely to breastfeed? *J Fam Pract, 51*(5), 431-436.

Tender, J. A. F., Janakiram, J., Arce, E., Mason, R., Jordan, T., Marsh, J., . . . Moon, R. Y. (2009). Reasons for in-hospital formula supplementation of breastfed infants from low-income families. *Journal of Human Lactation, 25*(1), 11-17.

Tinling, M. (2011). Senior Thesis. Environmental Sciences Department. UNC.

Truitt, S. T., Fraser, A. B., Grimes, D. A., Gallo, M. F., & Schulz, K. F. (2003). Combined hormonal versus nonhormonal versus progestin-only contraception in lactation. *Cochrane Database Syst Rev*(2), CD003988. doi: 10.1002/14651858.cd003988

U.S. Breastfeeding Committee. (2010). *Core competencies in breastfeeding care and services for all health professionals.* Retrieved December 14, 2012, from http://www.usbreastfeeding.org/Portals/0/Publications/Core-Competencies-2010-rev.pdf

U.S. Department of Health and Human Services. (2000). *HHS blueprint for action on breastfeeding.* Washington, D.C.: Office on Women's Health. Retrieved December 14, 2012 from http://www.womenshealth.gov/archive/breastfeeding/programs/

blueprints/bluprntbk2.pdf

U.S. Department of Health and Human Services. (2010). *Healthy People 2020 breastfeeding objectives.* Retrieved from: http://www.healthypeople.gov/2020/topicsobjectives2020/objectiveslist.aspx?topicid=26

U.S. Department of Health and Human Services. (2011). *The Surgeon General's call to action to support breastfeeding.* Washington, DC: Office of the Surgeon General, US Department of Health and Human Services. Retrieved from: http://www.surgeongeneral.gov/library/calls/breastfeeding/index.html

U.S. Department of Labor Wage and Hour Division. (2010). *Fact Sheet #73: Break Time for Nursing Mothers under the FLSA.* Retrieved from: http://www.dol.gov/whd/regs/compliance/whdfs73.htm#.UMtl0KX3BN0

U.S. Government Accountability Office. (2006). *Report to congressional addressees: Breastfeeding.* Retrieved from: http://www.gao.gov/new.items/d06282.pdf

UNICEF. (2012). *Childinfo. Monitoring the situation of children and women. Statistics by area / child nutrition.* Retrieved from: http://www.childinfo.org/breastfeeding_progress.html

UNICEF. (2012). *Nutrition: Infant and young child feeding and care: Protecting, promoting, and supporting breastfeeding.* Retrieved from: http://www.unicef.org/nutrition/index_breastfeeding.html

UNICEF. (2002). *State of the World's Children.* UNICEF, NY. Retrieved from: http://www.unicef.org/sowc/

UNICEF. (2005). *Celebrating the Innocenti Declaration on the protection, promotion and support of breastfeeding: Past achievements, present challenges and the way forward for infant and young child feeding.* UNICEF Innocenti Research Centre. Retrieved from: http://www.unicef.org/nutrition/files/Innocenti_plus15_BreastfeedingReport.pdf

UNICEF UK. (2012). *The Baby friendly initiative.* Retrieved from: http://www.unicef.org.uk/babyfriendly/

UNICEF/WHO. (1990). *Innocenti Declaration on the protection, promotion, and support of breastfeeding.* Retrieved from: http://www.unicef.org/programme/breastfeeding/innocenti.htm

United States Agency for International Development. (2012). *ADS Chapter 212: Breastfeeding Promotion: Functional Series 200 – Programming Policy.* Retrieved from: http://transition.usaid.gov/policy/ads/200/212.pdf

USBC. (2008). *Achieving exclusive breastfeeding in the United States: Findings and recommendations.* Washington, DC: United States Breastfeeding Committee. Retrieved from: http://www.usbreastfeeding.org/AboutUs/PublicationsPositionStatements/tabid/70/Default.aspx

Verma, M., Chhatwal, J., & Varughese, P. V. (1995). Antenatal period: An educational opportunity. *Indian Pediatr, 32*(2), 171-177.

Watkins, A. L., & Dodgson, J. E. (2010). Breastfeeding educational interventions for health professionals: A synthesis of intervention studies. *Journal for Specialists in Pediatric Nursing, 15*(3), 223-232.

Whalen, B., & Cramton, R. (2010). Overcoming barriers to breastfeeding continuation and exclusivity. *Current Opinion in Pediatrics, 22*(5), 655.

WHO/UNICEF. (1989). *Protecting, promoting and supporting breast-feeding: The special role of maternity services.* A joint WHO/UNICEF statement. Retrieved from: http://whqlibdoc.who.int/publications/9241561300.pdf

Witt, A. M., Smith, S., Mason, M. J., & Flocke, S. A. (2012). Integrating routine lactation consultant support into a pediatric practice. *Breastfeeding Medicine, 7*(1), 38-42.

World Health Organization. (1981). *International code of marketing of breast-milk substitutes.* Geneva, Switzerland.

World Health Organization. (2000-2004). Child and adolescent health and development: Infant and young child feeding: exclusive breastfeeding. Geneva: WHO.

World Health Organization. (2009). Medical eligibility criteria for contraceptive use. (4th ed.). Geneva, Swtizerland.

World Health Organization. Division of Diarrhoeal Acute Respiratory Disease Control. Working Group on Infant Feeding. (1991). *Indicators for Assessing Breast-feeding Practices: Report of an Informal Meeting, 11-12 June 1991.* Geneva, Switzerland: World Health Organization.

World Health Organization/UNICEF. (2003). *Global strategy for infant and young child feeding.* Retrieved from: http://whqlibdoc.who.int/publications/2003/9241562218.pdf

Wright, C. M., Parkinson, K., & Scott, J. (2006). Breast-feeding in a UK urban context: Who breast-feeds, for how long and does it matter? *Public Health Nutrition, 9*(6), 686-691.

Yarmo, K., & Malin, C. (2005). *Reaching minorty groups with culturally competent prenatal health education.* Paper presented at the 133rd Annual Meeting & Exposition of the American Public Health Association, Philidelphia, PA.

Zanardo, V., Svegliado, G., Cavallin, F., Giustardi, A., Cosmi, E., Litta, P., & Trevisanuto, D. (2010). Elective cesarean delivery: Does it have a negative effect on breastfeeding? *Birth, 37*(4), 275-279.

Index of Tables and Figures

Glossary of Acronyms and Abbreviations

ACA	Affordable Care Act
AAP	American Academy of Pediatrics
ABM	Academy of Breastfeeding Medicine
ANC	Antenatal care
BF	Breastfed/breastfeed/breastfeeding
CGBI	Carolina Global Breastfeeding Institute
C/S	Caesarean section
d(s)	Day(s)
DHHS	U.S. Department of Health and Human Services
EBF	Exclusively breastfed exclusively breastfeed/exclusive breastfeeding
FF	Formula fed/formula feed/formula feeding
GAO	United States Government Accountability Office
hr(s)	Hour(s)
HRSA	Health Resource Service Administration
IBCLC	International Board Certified Lactation Consultant
IBFAN	International Baby Food Action Network
LAM	Lactational Amenorrhea Method
LBW	Low birthweight
LC	Lactation Consultant, indicates IBCLC
LLLI	La Leche League, International
MCH	Maternal and Child Health
MCHB	Maternal and Child Health Bureau
mo(s)	Month(s)
NGO	Non-Governmental Organization
NICU	Neonatal Intensive Care Unit
OR	Odds ratio

OWH	Office of Women's Health
PBF	Predominant breastfeeding
pp	Postpartum
SBF	Sustained breastfeeding
SES	Socioeconomic status
sig.	Significant
UNC	University of North Carolina at Chapel Hill
UNICEF	United Nations Children's Fund
USBC	United Stated Breastfeeding Committee
USG	United States Government
VBAC	Vaginal Birth After Caesarean Section
WABA	World Alliance for Breastfeeding Action
w/	With
w/o	Without
WHO	World Health Organization
wk(s)	Week(s)
WIC	Special Supplemental Nutrition Program for Women, Infants, and Children
y.o.	Years old
yr(s)	Year(s)

Bibliography

For a summary of all references cited in the book, go to www.ibreastfeeding. com/chl12bibliography.

About the Authors

Miriam H. Labbok, MD, MPH, IBCLC, FACPM, FABM, FILCA

Professor – Department of Maternal and Child Health, Gillings School of Global Public Health, Chapel Hill, North Carolina

Director – Carolina Global Breastfeeding Institute

Dr. Labbok is dedicated to enabling all women to achieve their reproductive health intentions, with an emphasis on optimal breastfeeding, as well as birth and birth spacing, in an intergenerational approach to family health. She served as the Senior Advisor for Infant and Young Child Feeding and Care, UNICEF HQ, where she supported the *Innocenti+15* conference and oversaw the revision and updates on the BFHI approach and materials; Chief, Maternal Health and Nutrition, USAID; Director, Breastfeeding and Maternal Health, Institute for Reproductive Health, and Associate Professor, Georgetown University, where she played a key role in the development of the Lactational Amenorrhea Method for birth spacing; and Assistant Professor at Johns Hopkins School of Public Health. Her advisor in her MD-MPH training was Dr. Cicely Williams. A founder and past president of the Academy of Breastfeeding Medicine, leader in APHA International Health and Population Section work, and pediatric epidemiologist, she has served as an expert and/or consultant for the U.S. and NC Institutes of Medicine, the World Bank, Centers for Disease Control and Prevention, and WHO expert committees related to MCHN/FP, and serves on the U.S. Secretary of Health's Advisory Committee on Infant Mortality. With more than100 articles in refereed journals, more than 40 chapters and edited books, dozens of monographs, and hundreds of scientific presentations, her research, teaching, and service are dedicated to operational research and translation of research evidence into well evaluated service and social change activities. She has been honored for her work by USAID, LLLI, ILCA, all of her schools of higher learning, and other organizations.

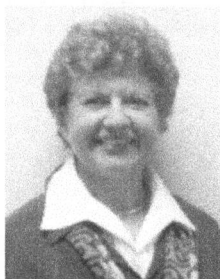

Emily C. Taylor, MPH, IHI-IA, LCCE, CD (DONA)

Deputy Director – Carolina Global Breastfeeding Institute, Department of Maternal and Child Health, Gillings School of Global Public Health, The University of North Carolina at Chapel Hill

Emily Taylor works to reduce socio-ecological constraints to breastfeeding in the United

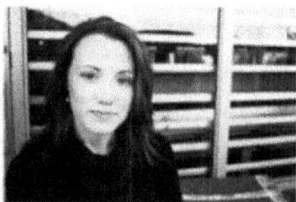

States with particular emphasis on healthcare delivery systems. She is responsible for Collaborative Quality Improvement facilitation with groups of hospitals in North Carolina, and works to help improve the quality of their maternity care services in hopes of increasing the number of women who meet their breastfeeding goals. Emily serves as the Secretary of the Board of the United States Breastfeeding Committee and the Chair of the North Carolina Breastfeeding Coalition. She is a Master of Public Health, an IHI Improvement Advisor, and a certified Leadership Facilitator. Though she no longer has an active practice, her experience as a childbirth doula and Lamaze educator continue to inform her practice.

Kathy Parry, MPH, IBCLC, LMBT, CEIM

Project Director — Carolina Global Breastfeeding Institute, Department of Maternal and Child Health, Gillings School of Global Public Health, The University of North Carolina at Chapel Hill

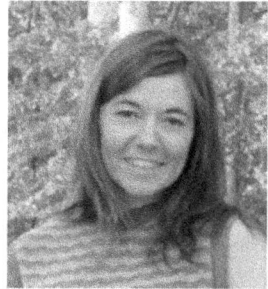

Kathy Parry joined CGBI in May of 2012 after two years as a graduate research assistant with the Institute. Her current work involves supporting and evaluating a prenatal breastfeeding education program currently being offered through UNC Health Care: Ready, Set Baby. Kathy also assisted in research on women's perceptions and reactions to infant formula advertisements. She is an internationally board certified lactation consultant and an active member of the North Carolina Breastfeeding Coalition. She is also a licensed prenatal massage therapist, with special interests in craniosacral therapy for infants and educating parents in the art of infant massage.